Critical Care Focus
12: The Psychological Challenges of Intensive Care

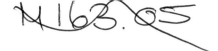

Critical Care Focus

12: The Psychological Challenges

of Intensive Care

EDITED BY
DR SAXON A RIDLEY
Consultant in Anaesthesia and Intensive Care
Norfolk and Norwich University Hospital
Colney Lane, Norwich, UK

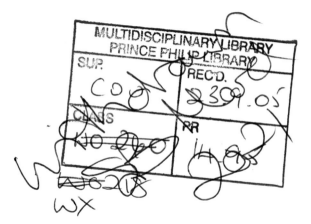

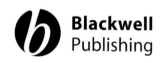

Blackwell
Publishing

© 2005 by Blackwell Publishing Ltd
BMJ Books is an imprint of the BMJ Publishing Group Limited, used under licence

Blackwell Publishing, Inc., 350 Main Street, Malden,
Massachusetts 02148-5020, USA
Blackwell Publishing Ltd, 9600 Garsington Road, Oxford OX4 2DQ, UK
Blackwell Publishing Asia Pty Ltd, 550 Swanston Street,
Carlton, Victoria 3053, Australia

First published 2005

Library of Congress Cataloging-in-Publication Data
The psychological challenges of intensive care / edited by Saxon A. Ridely.
p.; cm.—(Critical care focus; 12) ISBN 0-7279-1794-3.
1.   Critical Care medicine—Psychological aspects—Congresses.
2.   Catastrophic illness—Psychological aspects—Congresses.
[DLNM: 1.   Critical Care—psychology—Congresses.   2. Critical Illness—
psychology—Congresses.   3.   Stress, Psychological—Congresses. WX 218 P9737
2005]   I.   Ridley, Saxon.II. Intensive Care Society (Great
Britain)   III.   Title.   IV.   Series: Critical care focus series ; 12
RC86.7.p79   2005
616.02'8—dc22
2004020632

ISBN 0727917943

A catalogue record for this title is available from the British Library

Set in 10/12 MPlantin by Kolam Information Services Pvt. Ltd, Pondicherry, India
Printed and bound in India by Replika Press Pvt. Ltd

Commissioning Editor: Mary Banks
Development Editor: Claire Bonnett
Production Controller: Kate Charman

For further information on Blackwell Publishing, visit our website:
http://www.blackwellpublishing.com

Contents

CONTENTS

Critical Care Focus Series

Also available:

Contributors

Anetth Granberg Axèll
Senior Lecturer, University of Lund, Department of Nursing, Lund, Sweden

Carl G Bäckman
Senior Intensive Care Nurse, Department of Anaesthesia and Intensive Care, Vrinnevisjukhuset, Norrköping, Sweden

Stephen Brett
Consultant in Intensive Care, Department of Anaesthesia and Intensive Care, Hammersmith Hospital, Du Cane Road, London, UK

Gillian Colville
Consultant Clinical Psychologist, Paediatric Psychology Service, St George's Hospital, London, UK

Martin A Conway
Department of Psychology, University of Durham, Science Laboratories, Durham, UK

Brian H Cuthbertson
Clinical Senior Lecturer in Anaesthesia and Intensive Care, Medicine and Therapeutics, Institute of Medical Sciences, University of Aberdeen, Foresterhill, Aberdeen, UK

Richard D Griffiths
Professor of Medicine, Intensive Care Research Group, Department of Medicine, Duncan Building, UCD, University of Liverpool, Liverpool, UK

Alastair Hull
Consultant Psychiatrist, Murray Royal Hospital, Muirhall Road, Perth, Scotland, UK

Christina Jones
Consultant Nurse Critical Care Follow-up, Intensive Care Unit, Whiston Hospital, Merseyside, UK

Carl S Waldmann
Consultant in Anaesthesia and Intensive Care Medicine, Intensive Care Unit, Royal Berkshire Hospital, Reading, UK

Sten M Walther
Director of Intensive Care, Department of Anaesthesia and Intensive Care, University Hospital, Örebro, Sweden

Preface to the Critical Care Focus Series

The Critical Care Focus Series aims to provide a snapshot of current thought and practice, by renowned experts. The complete series should provide a comprehensive guide for all health professionals on key issues in today's field of critical care. The volumes are deliberately concise and easy to read, designed to inform and provoke. Most chapters are produced from transcriptions of lectures given at the Intensive Care Society meetings and represent the views of world leaders in their fields.

Saxon Ridley

Introduction

This, the twelfth volume in the Critical Care Focus series, concentrates on the psychological consequences of critical illness. It comprises transcripts of lectures delivered by internationally renowned experts at the Intensive Care Society's Focus Meeting held in February 2004. The lectures concentrate on this often-neglected aspect of patient care.

Chapter 1 reviews the disturbances of memory that are likely to arise following critical care admission. Episode memory is classified as primary (short-term) or secondary (long-term). The disorders of episodic memory are classified as anterograde or retrograde amnesia. Such amnesia is frequently seen in brain-injured patients but can also occur after critical care. These disorders may result in intrusive memories that contribute to post-traumatic stress reactions.

Chapter 2 discusses the consequences and the ripple effect of trauma. The normal reactions to a traumatic experience are discussed. Post-traumatic stress disorder (PTSD) is common, and is a recognised clinical entity. However, there are well-recognised risk factors for developing PTSD and these relate to the trauma itself, the patient (genetic predisposition, cortisol response and gender) and the environment including the intensive care unit (ICU). Treatment is based on the early recognition of the disorder, followed by the application of well-recognised psychological therapies.

Chapter 3 offers an insight into what must be a confusing and frightening time for patients. It describes the ICU experience from the patients' perspective by giving their feelings and reactions to severe illness and the treatment they receive.

Chapter 4 outlines the pathophysiological basis of the delirium that can occur in critically ill patients while on the ICU. Delirium can be quantitatively assessed using the Confusion Assessment Method for ICU. Frequently, delirium is caused by encephalopathy, and the psychological problems seen may be related to structural changes in the brain. The effective management of delirium requires care both in and after intensive care unit admission.

Chapter 5 briefly discusses the therapeutic approaches to the significant psychological stress in both the relatives and the patients. After discharge, anxiety and depression are common and the levels of such symptoms are predictive of PTSD development. The diagnostic criteria for PTSD are well recognised. The basis for the PTSD is discussed in terms of the cognitive and neuro-circuitry models.

Chapter 6 presents and reviews results of work carried out at St George's Hospital on the impact of admission to paediatric ICUs. Intensive care admission for a child can be extremely traumatic for both the parents and child. The literature on the parents' experiences on paediatric ICUs is limited. Recent advances have shown that the children may also suffer extreme stress reactions.

Chapter 7 outlines the methods and results of cognitive testing following critical illness. Critical illness affects all the major organ systems of the body, including the brain. Cognitive dysfunction is common after anaesthesia and surgery, but appears to be even more pronounced following a critical illness. A manifestation of this cognitive impairment is the psychological repercussions following ICU admission.

Chapter 8 outlines how, by keeping a contemporaneous photo diary of the patients while they are on intensive care, autobiographical data may be used to help them recover from the psychological and physical consequences of their admission. Loss of this information could be one of the most stressful aspects of ICU admission. The author includes some fascinating examples of patients' stories and extracts from their photo diaries.

Chapter 9 outlines the stresses that make working in a critical care environment difficult. Working in critical care is recognised to be stressful. Unfortunately, particularly in the United Kingdom, human resources management and conditions at work do not capitalise on the staff's potential.

1: Disorders of episodic memory

MARTIN A CONWAY

Introduction

This chapter reviews disturbances of memory and considers those likely to arise following a period of treatment in an intensive care unit (ICU). Obviously there are many factors that influence a patient's memory while on ICU. These include the nature, severity and duration of illness, suddenness of onset, period of delirium, effects of drugs, mechanical ventilation, and the unusual and unfamiliar environment of the ICU. In some patients, these may lead to amnesia while in others, to memories that lack specificity. At the opposite pole, critical illness may induce a powerful stress response leading to post-traumatic stress disorder (PTSD) or a subset of PTSD symptoms. After ICU, patients may have vivid highly intrusive memories of emotionally destabilising experiences that cause intense anxiety and distress. The implications of these and other memory disturbances for mental well-being after ICU are briefly considered.

Disturbances of memory, often as intense as those seen in psychiatric illnesses, can arise as a consequence, sometimes a secondary consequence, of many different types of medical intervention. For instance, any procedure in which blood flow to the brain is attenuated or interrupted will affect critical brain structures that are essential for normal memory. The hippocampal formation in the medial temporal lobes (part of a system known as the 'medial temporal lobe' (MTL) memory system [1,2]) is especially vulnerable to falls in blood oxygen levels and is a structure that rapidly degrades in anoxic episodes. Because the MTL is crucial for encoding new information into long-term memory, damage to the hippocampus and related structures often results in a specific form of amnesia (such as anterograde amnesia, which is the reduction in, or loss of, the ability to encode new information). There are many other disturbances of memory that can follow general medical experiences. However, it may be useful to review the different sorts of memory and types of long-term knowledge identified by memory researchers.

Memory types

A major distinction, made over a hundred years ago by William James [3], is the division of memory into short-term or primary memory and long-term or secondary memory. Short-term memory has a limited capacity of about five to nine items ('items' can be pretty much anything from thoughts, images, words and numbers). It also has a limited duration of about a couple of minutes. In most forms of amnesia short-term memory is undamaged, and this is probably because the neural networks that mediate this complicated system are distributed over several brain areas, especially the prefrontal cortex. Thus, paradoxically and disturbingly, patients with dense antero-grade amnesia, due to brain damage or some more intermittent influence (e.g. the effects of a drug), would be able to hold a conversation but after about 2 min would not be able to recall to whom or about what they were talking. In recent work the term 'short-term' memory has been largely replaced by the concept of 'working memory' [4,5,6]. Working memory captures the idea that short-term retention is not simply some sort of passive memory store but rather a complicated amalgam of several different types of knowledge (e.g. auditory, visual, haptic, affective), transitorily configured into a dynamic mental model [7] that represents the current processing sequence in all its complexity. It is important to note that only a small part of this ever enters conscious awareness. This is achieved by executive processes (in the prefrontal cortex) that coordinate the underlying knowledge networks, which at any one time mediate the current processing sequence and which we experience as 'the stream of consciousness'.

Long-term memory is a very different system, which has features and properties that are the opposite of short-term or working memory. For example, the capacity of long-term memory is not known but is, by all estimates, considered to be extremely large. Think, for example, of the tens of thousands of words an adult can bring to mind and use, the thousands of facts, the vast range of actions, and of course the one thing that we are all experts on – memory for our own lives (autobiographical memory). Similarly, duration of knowledge in long-term memory is measured in hours, days, weeks, months, years, decades and lifetimes rather than seconds and minutes. Some researchers have argued that nothing is ever actually forgotten or lost; instead what happens is that access to long-term knowledge is lost but that knowledge nonetheless remains available in memory and can in principle still be accessed. Indeed, inaccessible knowledge might still influence experience and behaviour non-consciously. Consider, for example, a patient who underwent a traumatic medical experience but was amnesic of it. This patient might nonetheless experience considerable anxiety if a similar situation were to arise. The view that nothing is ever forgotten is, however, a fairly extreme hypothesis and what is more likely is that some things are forgotten while others are not. For example, even in advanced old age the meanings of words are not forgotten (although they can be in pathological ageing such as semantic dementia [8]) and many concepts are retained in full. One does not forget basic actions like shaving or brushing one's hair and vivid experiences may be consistently recalled. On the other hand, name-finding difficulties do increase with age and executive processes become less efficient. Memories may fossilise with retelling and rethinking into mental representations that resemble stories rather than 'live' image-based affect-laden memories.

In addition to the basic distinction between working memory and long-term memory, researchers have made important distinctions between knowledge types in long-term memory. Three of these are procedural memory, semantic memory and episodic memory. Procedural memory typically refers to motor programs that mediate actions. This type of knowledge is not consciously accessible. Thus, most people could, if requested, whistle the national anthem, but in doing so there would be no conscious access to knowledge and procedures that mediate this behaviour. Interestingly in disorders such as amnesia, procedural knowledge is intact (e.g. amnesics do not forget how to brush their hair, shave, whistle or ride bicycles) and some learning of new skills is also possible. Semantic and episodic long-term knowledge are different, being 'declarative' rather than 'procedural'. Thus, for example, one can consciously recall that 'Paris is the capital of France' (a semantic concept) and remember staying in a hotel in Paris' Latin quarter many years ago (a type of episodic memory sometimes referred to as 'autobiographical' memory). There is, however, the possibility of some confusion. Autobiographical memories invariably involve auto-biographical factual or conceptual knowledge (e.g. the individual visiting Paris) in conjunction with episodic memories. Episode memories are 'experience near', derived from working memory, and, in human memory, predominantly in the form of visual images. Episodic memories represent highly specific knowledge of single experiences and contain sensory-perceptual and affective–conceptual knowledge derived directly from actual experience. They provide crucial information for the self and identity, and form an important part of the 'content' of the self. Episodic memories tie the self into a record of a lived, personal, history and in so doing they determine the nature of the individual in the present, as well as provide a basis for future planning (see [9,10,11] for extended accounts of autobiographical and episodic memory). These inherently psychological representations of past experience (i.e. episodic memories) are contextualised by semantic conceptual knowledge but stand separately from it.

Disorders of episodic memory

Disorders of episodic memory include amnesia, intrusive memories, memory specificity and distorted and false memories. It seems that many, if not all of these, occur to some degree in patients who have experience of ICU. Jones [12] provides a detailed and comprehensive review of memory disorders in ICU patients.

Amnesia

Amnesia has two forms: anterograde and retrograde. Anterograde amnesia is a reduction in, or complete loss of, the ability to encode new information and especially to form new episodic memories. Anterograde amnesia has multiple causes, such as closed and open head injuries, viral infections, tumour, anoxia and drug overdose. The extent that these impact on limbic system circuits determines the anterograde amnesia density. It is important to note that in the majority of amnesic patients, including anterograde amnesia patients, premorbid levels of intellect and short-term working memory remain intact. Moreover, even patients with dense anterograde amnesia often have a relatively intact autobiographical memory for their life prior to their injury even though they may have no enduring memory of subsequent events.

Retrograde amnesia refers to loss of episodic memories predating the onset of illness. It is very rare to encounter retrograde amnesia on its own when it is known as 'focal retrograde amnesia'. Instead retrograde amnesia in brain-damaged patients is combined with at least some degree of anterograde amnesia (which often indicates hippocampal lesions). Retrograde amnesia rarely if ever encompasses the whole premorbid period (which is the 'Hollywood' concept of retrograde amnesia). Retrograde amnesia varies in its density. Often it is temporally graded, stretching back for a few minutes or longer after injury. Typically, access to memories dating from late adolescence and childhood events is preserved. These are often the last memories to be lost in advanced stages of dementia and seem especially resistant to loss of access, perhaps because of their centrality to self. Islands of memory are occasionally preserved but memory is fragmented and its temporal order may be disrupted or lost.

Patients who have been in ICU very frequently have retrograde amnesia for their ICU stay with preservation of some memory fragments [12]. There are many causes of retrograde amnesia in ICU patients such as delirium, critical illness itself and drugs. However, delirium may be the most important. Delirium powerfully and negatively impacts on the complex configural process of working memory [5] and is experienced by the patient as degradation and break up of the 'stream of consciousness'. A complicated, continuously evolving mental model of the present cannot be generated, and instead, only fragmentary memories of the present are possible and these may lack meaning. Assuming that encoding of episodic memories is still possible under these circumstances, the resulting memories reflect the malfunctioning of working memory during delirium.

However, the situation is almost certainly compounded by intermittent malfunction of the MTL (which contains networks vital for encoding). This may arise because the disturbing experience of reality during delirium is traumatic for the patient and the trauma causes a stress response. In this response, blood sugar levels are raised and brain glucocorticoids increase. The effect of this is to overstimulate hippocampal networks and so impair or prevent encoding. Indeed, permanent reductions in hippocampal volume have been reliably found in trauma survivors (see [13] for a review) and this occurs due to the increase of glucocorticoid neurohormones to chronically high levels. Thus, delirium and the hormonal effects lead to the encoding of highly disrupted trauma-like memory containing enigmatic visual images and distorted comprehension of experience.

Intrusive memories

Traumatic experiences often give rise to vivid memories of specific moments of trauma. These are emotionally debilitating and can incapacitate the patient with intense feelings of anxiety and/or guilt. In PTSD the intrusive recall of traumatic memories is one of the prominent symptoms. Intrusive recall and the associated disturbances of affect are so frequent and intense in PTSD that they can lead to severe disruption of daily activities with marked attempts to avoid anything that reminds the patients of their traumatic experience (see [14] for a recent review). However, PTSD memories are not accurate or full records of the trauma. They can be distorted and may even contain wholly false details [15]. Initially, they are often disordered and fragmentary without the conceptual and thematic knowledge that provides an organising structure. Treatment involves reliving (e.g. recalling the memories during therapy), overcoming distortions and errors, correcting temporal distortions and developing a more conceptually structured set of memories.

Patients who have been in ICU appear to suffer from something like PTSD [12]. In many patients this may not approach the full PTSD syndrome but in others a full PTSD illness may result. Indeed, many ICU patients have intrusive memories, often of paranoid fantasies and hallucinations. These may arise from hallucinations of delirium, from the effects of drugs, fatigue, as well as from their own physical illness, especially when brain blood flow is reduced or where there is a stress response leading to a surge in glucocorticoid levels. Other groups prone to PTSD are soldiers who have taken part in active combat, rape victims, victims of violence, road traffic accidents and other accident survivors and people (including children) who have been physically, sexually and/or emotionally abused. PTSD symptoms have been observed in children as young as 5 years, and work has been undertaken on children's memories for painful medical procedures (but not on any procedure quite as extreme as ICU organ

5

support). It should be noted that a PTSD reaction to trauma can remain dormant for many years and then reappear. Delayed PTSD in World War II veterans has been observed and it might be that with age-related changes to memory (especially those arising from changes to the frontal lobes), previously inhibited PTSD is allowed expression. Moreover, encountering a powerful cue that activates inhibited or avoided PTSD memories may also initiate the syndrome and the sudden onset of intrusive recollections.

Memory specificity

In many psychological illnesses, episodic memories are apparently difficult to access and instead the individual recalls general events (e.g. walking in the park rather than a specific memory of one particular walk in the park). General memories are characteristic of clinical levels of depression [16] where they may serve a defensive function (e.g. prevent access of painful, traumatic, memories). They have also been observed in schizophrenics, obsessive–compulsive patients, in neurological patients with frontal lobe damage and in the very elderly. One problem with general memories is that they do not provide the specificity needed for future planning, nor do they effectively anchor the self in personal history and so allow wishful aspects of personality and self more expression. The incidence of depression in ICU patients is not known but will be higher than that in the normal population simply because depression is a common reaction to life stress. Indeed, it has been called the 'common cold' of mental disorders. Thus, some ICU patients may have what appear to be rather general low-specificity memories for their time in the ICU and, quite possibly, for the preceding and following events.

Distorted and false memories

Distorted and false memories occur following trauma, delirium and damage to certain brain areas, especially the frontal lobes (when they are known as 'confabulations'). Confabulations can be especially disturbing both for the patient and for friends and relatives. The sisters of one patient with frontal lobe damage complained of her constant 'lying' after her physical recovery from a road traffic accident. Confabulations can take the forms of 'honest lies' [17] and present plausible accounts of events that did not in fact take place. They also take more fantastic forms. For example, Jones provides an illustrative case of a patient who, while in the ICU, suffered from the Capgras' delusion that her family had been replaced by aliens. The subsequent intrusive false memory was so convincing that she declined any further surgery. Fantastic confabulations and probably more frequent but harder to detect plausible confabulations may be fairly common in memories of ICU experiences. However, the incidence is unknown. More effective communication with ICU patients might reduce the incidence of confabulations.

Disorders of memory awareness

These occur in epilepsy, temporal lobe pathology, delirium, and perhaps in very old age. Recollective experience, the sense of the self in the past, is one way in which the brain can indicate that remembering is taking place, rather than imagining, fantasising or daydreaming. Research suggests that this 'feeling of remembering' may be mediated by circuits in the temporal lobe [15]. When these malfunction they may trigger recollective experience for mental states other than remembering. This seems to happen in the 'dream' state that precedes seizure onset in temporal lobe epilepsy. It may also occur in older patients with temporal lobe pathology who suffer chronic and persistent experiences of *déjà vécu* (the experience of having lived through the present moment before while *déjà vu*, in contrast, is the experience of having seen something before); patients may act on their experiences of *déjà vécu* [18]. Disorders of recollection or of the feeling of remembering are a relatively new area of study and may be under-reported. It would be unusual to complain of repeated feelings of having lived through the recent moment before (and we have detected only two patients referred for 'persistent déjà vu').

Conclusion

Extreme experiences that involve delirium, unusual physical experiences, drugs and intense negative emotions give rise in many people to disturbed memories. In some the result may be amnesia and other general memories. In others the effect may be full PTSD or PTSD-like mental illness. In all patients we need to determine the incidence of these negative reactions, understand their causes and develop effective intervention and treatment programs.

References

1. Moscovitch M. Memory and working-with-memory: a component process model based on modules and central systems. *J Cog Neurosci* 1992;4:257–67.
2. Squire LR. Memory and the hippocampus: a synthesis from findings with rats, monkeys, and humans. *Psych Rev* 1992;**99**:195–231.
3. James W. *The Principles of Psychology*. New York: Holt, Rinehart & Winston. 1890.

4. Baddeley AD. *Working Memory*. Oxford: Clarendon Press, 1986.
5. Baddeley AD. The episodic buffer: a new component of working memory? *Trends Cog Sci* 2000;4:417–23.
6. Baddeley AD, Hitch GJ. Working memory. In: Bower GA, ed. *The Psychology of Learning and Motivation*. New York: Academic Press, 1974, pp. 47–89.
7. Johnson-Laird PN. *Mental Models: Toward a Cognitive Science of Language, Inference, and Consciousness*. Cambridge: Cambridge University Press, 1983.
8. Hodges JR. Memory in the dementias. In: Tulving E, Craik FIM, eds. *The Oxford Handbook of Human Memory*. Oxford: Oxford University Press, 2000, pp. 441–63.
9. Conway MA, Pleydell-Pearce CW. The construction of autobiographical memories in the self memory system. *Psych Rev* 2000;107:261–88.
10. Conway MA. Sensory perceptual episodic memory and its context: autobiographical memory. *Phil Trans R Soc Lond* 2001;B 356:1375–84.
11. Conway MA, Singer JA, Tagini A. The self and autobiographical memory: correspondence and coherence. *Social Cognition* 2004;22:495–537.
12. Jones C, Griffiths RD, Humphris G. Disturbed memory and amnesia related to intensive care. *Memory* 2000;8:79–94.
13. Conway MA, Fthenaki A. Disruption and loss of autobiographical memory. In: Cermak LS, ed. *Handbook of Neuropsychology, Memory and Its Disorders*, 2nd edn. Amsterdam: Elsevier, 2000, pp. 281–312.
14. Ehlers A, Hackmann A, Michael T. Intrusive reexperiencing in posttraumatic stress disorder: phenomenology, theory, and therapy. *Memory* 2004; 12:403–15.
15. Conway MA, Meares K, Standart S. Images and goals. *Memory* 2004; 12:525–31.
16. Williams JMG. Depression and the specificity of autobiographical memory. In: Rubin DC, ed. *Remembering Our Past: Studies in Autobiographical Memory*. Cambridge: Cambridge University Press, 1996, pp. 244–67.
17. Moscovitch M. Confabulation and the frontal systems: strategic versus associative retrieval in neuropsychological theories of memory. In: Roediger HL III, Craik FIM, eds. *Varieties of Memory and Consciousness: Essays in Honour of Endel Tulving*. Hillsdale, NJ: Lawrence Erlbaum Associates, 1989, pp. 133–60.
18. Moulin JAC, Conway MA, Thompson R, James N, Jones RW. Disordered memory awareness: recollective confabulation in two cases of persistent déjà vu. *Neuropsychologia* 2005 (in press).

2: Life interrupted: risk factors for post-traumatic reactions

ALASTAIR M HULL, BRIAN H CUTHBERTSON

Introduction

Surviving a major disaster or suffering extensive burns is readily identifiable as a severe traumatic event that may precipitate acute psychological distress and subsequent chronic psychological morbidity. However, more common traumatic events such as road traffic accidents, assaults, workplace trauma and life-threatening illness can also lead to psychological morbidity. Patients with physical injury such as burns or facial trauma have been studied. However, recently researchers have demonstrated post-traumatic psychological sequelae, such as post-traumatic stress disorder (PTSD), after critical illness and thereby highlighted the need to recognise these disorders.

Whilst some traumatic events appear so inherently awful that they cause high rates of post-traumatic reactions, it should be remembered that no traumatic event leads invariably to a psychological disorder. Indeed, individuals demonstrate remarkable resilience, and clinicians should not 'pathologise' what is often a process of normal adjustment rather than illness. Research has identified characteristics that predispose individuals to develop post-traumatic psychomorbidity. In this chapter we will highlight risk factors identified by epidemiological studies, the examination of specific clinical trauma populations and from critically ill patients. We will also discuss features of both 'normal' and pathological reactions to traumatic events and give an overview of the treatment options available.

The nature of traumatic events

People are exposed to traumatic events either in communities (e.g. disasters) or individually. Individual exposure can be further split into *intentional* (e.g. assault, robbery or rape) or *unintentional* (e.g. motor vehicle accident, industrial accident, medical event or related to critical illness). Traumatic events affect not just those directly involved but also those witnessing or confronted by the event, the so-called *ripple effect* of trauma. Within current classification systems [1,2] (DSM-IV; ICD-10), the traumatic event is viewed as the primary and overriding causal factor for post-traumatic conditions such as PTSD. However, as detailed below, this may not be entirely correct.

Normal reactions to traumatic experience or severe stress

Community studies have shown that two-thirds of people experiencing a traumatic event will have a normal acute response and will not develop subsequent psychological sequelae. Common early normal reactions to trauma include fear, numbness and denial, depression, anger, guilt, helplessness, hopelessness, sleep problems, hyperarousal, hypervigilance, perceptual changes (particularly in time) and flashbacks [3]. Occasionally elation may occur, as a result of having survived. The majority of patients can be reassured that their reactions are normal. Clinically, normal and pathological reactions are distinguished by their severity and duration. For example, the consensus statement on PTSD from the International Consensus Group on Depression and Anxiety [4] suggests starting a non-benzodiazepine hypnotic (such as zolpidem or zopiclone) for insomnia if sleep disturbance is present for four consecutive nights after trauma.

Pathological reactions to traumatic experience

Potential psychological reactions range from acute reactions such as acute stress disorder or grief reactions to chronic disorders such as depression, agoraphobia, alcohol and/or drug dependence, panic disorder, specific phobias (e.g. travel phobia) and PTSD. In a study of road traffic accident survivors aged 17–69 years without serious physical injury, Mayou *et al.* [3] found 19% had an anxiety disorder, 15% PTSD, 15% phobic travel anxiety and 6% a mood disorder at 1 year. For those with serious injury the figures were 19%, 28%, 28% and 8% respectively.

Post-traumatic stress disorder

PTSD is almost unique amongst psychiatric disorders because it includes an aetiological factor, the stressor (i.e. the traumatic event), as one of its core criteria. The event is accepted as 'traumatic' if it provokes an emotional reaction (comprising fear, helplessness or horror) and is perceived to have threatened serious injury or death. Notably, it is the individual's subjective experience of threat rather than the clinician's view that is important. Whilst there are many potential symptoms incorporated into post-traumatic reactions, the core symptoms of PTSD are grouped into intrusive phenomena, avoidance and numbing phenomena and hyperarousal symptoms (Table 2.1).

PTSD usually has an early onset with symptoms appearing within a few weeks, but fortunately for many patients the disorder may also resolve within 3 months. If symptoms are present at 3 months, they are likely to persist for much longer. PTSD may also be complicated by alcohol or drug misuse, often as a form of self-medicating. PTSD is readily identifiable but because of comorbidity and the overlap with symptoms of depression and other anxiety disorders, the diagnosis is easily missed unless the traumatic event is specifically asked about. In an intensive care setting, critical illness and its treatment should be acknowledged as a potential traumatic experience. In particular, avoidance of reminders is a symptom of PTSD, and thus patients may not volunteer this information unless prompted. Also, people believe 'time is a great healer' and may think their psychological symptoms are entirely normal and will settle eventually. Whilst time will allow resolution for some, it will allow the development of a chronic PTSD in others. There is no single diagnostic test for PTSD, and assessment must be conducted sensitively as trauma victims can find it hard to put their experience into words; too forceful an approach can lead to further trauma. It is helpful to reassure patients that an exhaustive description is not needed.

Whilst the characteristic symptoms of PTSD can be present shortly after the triggering event, the diagnosis requires the persistence of symptoms for 1 month, as well as significant impact on the level of functioning. Potential symptoms include suicidal thoughts, survivor guilt and dissociation.

Table 2.1 Core symptoms of post-traumatic stress disorder

Intrusive phenomena	Avoidant and emotional numbing symptoms	Hyperarousal symptoms
Recurrent distressing recollections	Avoiding reminders	Sleep disturbance
Nightmares	Avoiding thinking or talking about the event	Irritability/anger
Flashbacks (in any sensory modality)	Psychogenic amnesia	Concentration difficulties
Distress with reminders	Loss of interest	Hypervigilance
Physiological reactions (fight or flight)	Detachment Emotional numbing Sense of foreshortened future	Exaggerated startle response

In addition, it is important to identify comorbid conditions such as depression, anxiety disorders and alcohol or drug misuse.

PTSD is not the only possible psychological disorder after trauma and may not even be the most common as highlighted by Mayou's study [3]. Recent studies in the USA report the lifetime prevalence of PTSD at 8–12% [5]; however, prevalence rates have varied from 1% to 12.3% depending upon the methodology of the survey. It remains unclear how these findings can be translated to other populations; for example, no community survey has yet been completed in the UK.

It is important to identify those at risk of developing PTSD due to the often long-term disease burden; the average duration of an episode of PTSD is 7 years [5]. Individuals with PTSD have, for example, increased rates of cardiovascular, gastrointestinal and neurological and immunological symptoms. Individuals with PTSD also make greater use of the health services, have increased psychosomatic complaints and demonstrate an increased frequency of adverse health behaviours such as smoking, alcohol and drug misuse and risk-taking behaviour.

Risk factors for post-traumatic reactions

PTSD was initially regarded as a normal reaction to overwhelming stress. Primacy was given to the traumatic event with the trauma being seen as enough to cause the disorder without the need for vulnerability or risk factors. This was an attempt to distance PTSD from its inaccurate historical perception as resulting from 'moral inferiority' or inherent weakness. Research has now shown that PTSD is a biologically distinct entity and that risk factors are important in its development.

Whilst the relative weighting of aetiological risk factors for psychological disorders after trauma is not known, research has shown that outcome is a complex interaction among features of the trauma, the patient and the patient's environment. For example, the experience of a previous trauma may increase the risk of PTSD (i.e. sensitise the individual) but it may also inoculate if the individual believes he or she coped well with the previous trauma or critical illness.

Selected trauma populations have been studied in more depth and some prevalence rates are shown in Table 2.2. It is worth noting that the traumatic event has a 'ripple effect' affecting not just the victim but witnesses or rescuers also.

Vulnerability plays a significant role in who develops PTSD and whether it becomes a chronic disorder. However, no specific factors can explain the onset or course of PTSD. The most severe trauma does not lead invariably to the development of a psychological disorder. Some factors have been shown to have comparatively uniform predictive value for PTSD across trauma populations, whereas others have varying predictive value depend-

Table 2.2 Prevalence rates for different traumatic events

Trauma type	Prevalence rates (%)
Vietnam combat veterans [6]	15 (19 years after combat exposure)
Falklands War veterans [7]	22
Civil violence [8]	23
Major flood [9]	44
Road traffic accidents [4]	15
Rape of women [10]	35
Maxillofacial trauma [11]	41
ICU patients [12,13,14,15]	14–41
Major burns [16]	8–45
Major neurotrauma [17]	42 (6 months after trauma)
ICU after cardiac surgery [18]	18

ing upon the trauma population. Therefore, whilst findings from other populations are valuable, generalising findings from one trauma population to another should be undertaken with caution.

Trauma related risk factors

Trauma-related factors that affect vulnerability often possess intuitive validity. For example, prognosis is worse for survivors of 'man-made' rather than 'natural' events such as a flood because of issues like responsibility or malice. Further, if the trauma is sudden or unexpected, risk is increased. It has been suggested that this is due to the individual having no time to prepare. This may have great significance in an intensive care population. Further factors include prolonged exposure to the threat. This has commonly been seen to include being trapped or held hostage, and lengthy exposure in the form of prolonged ventilation has also been shown to be associated with post-traumatic psychomorbidity [12]. Other risk factors include threat to life as perceived by the victim (rather than by the clinician), multiple deaths and/or mutilation and personally relevant factors such as the involvement of a child, or identification with the victim or family. In addition, a dose-response relationship has been shown between the severity of the trauma and the likelihood of developing PTSD [19].

Patient related risk factors

There is a wide variety of patient-related risk factors for PTSD and the weighting of each factor is unknown. For example, previous trauma may either 'sensitise' or 'inoculate' the individual depending upon his or her view of the previous trauma experience. Furthermore, if the trauma causes physical injury, psychological outcome reflects the patient's perception of the seriousness of the injury rather than that of the surgeon [20].

Patient-related factors such as family or personal history of psychiatric disorder and previous childhood trauma (especially reported childhood abuse) have been found to be predictive across all trauma populations. Klein and colleagues have shown that in an orthopaedic trauma population the endorsement of the statement 'visited a GP for stress/distress' prior to the accident is a more reliable predictor than asking about pre-trauma psychiatric history [21]. Our study confirmed that endorsement of this statement was predictive of post-traumatic psychopathology (including PTSD) in an intensive care population [12]. Previous adult trauma predicts PTSD in some populations but not in others and demonstrates the complexity of this area. It has also been shown that certain coping styles and personality traits, such as being especially anxious prior to the trauma, are risk factors. For example, someone with a coping style typified by a belief of being in charge of their own destiny will have lower risk than someone who feels reliant on others.

Individuals at the extremes of age have been shown to be at greater risk of PTSD. Other patient-related risk factors include behavioural problems before 15 years of age (including truancy, vandalism and enuresis), lower educational, intelligence and socio-economic levels and a lifestyle with higher risk of traumatic events. The role of race had not yet been examined effectively with present epidemiological studies defining individuals dichotomously either as 'white' or 'non-white' [22].

Genetics

Though not yet replicated, neuroimaging has suggested pre-trauma smaller hippocampi may predispose an individual for PTSD [23]. This study examined monozygotic twins and found both trauma-exposed individuals with PTSD and their co-twins with neither a history of trauma nor psychomorbidity to have smaller hippocampi. This is significant, as hippocampal atrophy has been regularly reported in neuroimaging of subjects who have developed PTSD [24]. Other genetic findings include psychological characteristics that predispose to risk-taking behaviour. Genetic susceptibility has been shown to be only partially shared with risk for trauma exposure. In addition, there may be transgenerational effects as children of holocaust survivors (with PTSD) have both a higher risk of developing PTSD and lower cortisol levels [25,26].

Cortisol

Acute stress causes an increase in cortisol levels but the rise in cortisol levels is lowest in PTSD [27]. Lower cortisol levels in PTSD may represent an aberrant response or a vulnerability factor prior to trauma. Researchers have shown that cortisol levels are low at time of road traffic trauma in those later developing PTSD [28,29], and cortisol levels have been found to be low in rape victims with a previous history of rape or assault [30]. Chronic PTSD is characterised by low serum cortisol levels highlighting that PTSD is quantifiably separate from the stress response; it is not a normal response to an abnormal situation [31].

Gender

The role of gender remains unclear but epidemiological studies have suggested a role for gender in the development of PTSD. Males have been shown to be at greater risk of exposure to trauma whilst females are more likely to develop PTSD [5] after trauma exposure. However, other researchers have suggested gender may not have a role in vulnerability other than indirectly through the type of trauma people are exposed to, in particular violent sexual assault [31].

Post-traumatic risk factors

Post-traumatic risk factors include experiencing profound hopelessness and powerlessness, loss of normal daily function, such as employment [32], and suffering serious physical injury. The seriousness of the injury, in terms of psychological outcome, relates to the patient's perception rather than the clinician's [33]. Individuals who develop PTSD are more likely to have had a severe acute stress reaction, with dissociative experiences such as 'out-of-body experiences' that are rarely volunteered.

Environment related risk factors

Environmental factors that have been shown to act as risk factors for PTSD include lack of a support network (or the inability to utilise it), ongoing life stresses, the reaction of others and economic circumstances.

ICU-related risk factors

Studies of a range of trauma populations have shown that physical injuries are associated with psychological reactions such as PTSD. Psychological symptoms have been shown to occur commonly in different cohorts of critically ill patients. However, few studies of psychological outcome have examined factors associated with the development of PTSD. The risk factors that have been demonstrated in critical care populations are age (inversely) [12,15], gender (females more at risk than males) [15] and days of ventilation [12]. Intensive care unit length of stay and acute physiological assessment and chronic health evaluation (APACHE II) score were not risk factors for the development of PTSD in one cohort [12]. In this study, endorsement of the statement 'visited a GP or mental health professional for stress/psychological distress prior to the illness' was associated with a diagnosis of PTSD [12]. This reinforces the predictive value of previous history of mental distress or illness. Empirical studies of critical care populations have shown that the memory of trauma has a significant role though none have yet been replicated. For example, Jones and colleagues found that the absence of memory for real events in the intensive care unit (ICU) was associated with the development of PTSD [13] whilst Stoll and colleagues found the number of traumatic memories from ICU was associated with PTSD development [18].

Treatment

Staff in ICUs should not underestimate their role in the psychological care of trauma victims, as an early response may influence how the patient subsequently adjusts to the experience. Mental health specialists have an obvious role but this should not replace or overshadow the role of the intensive care staff or others such as family, friends or the clergy. As with other patient groups the provision of accurate and understandable information will be helpful but they should not be overloaded with this too early. Critical care staff will also have a crucial role in assessing the impact upon partner and family. There is also a need to target interventions towards those needing help, and let 'sleeping dogs lie' for those who are adjusting appropriately.

There is a growing number of empirically proven treatments for PTSD though there remains no 'gold standard'. There is no psychotropic medication of choice but there is increasing evidence supporting the use of serotonergic antidepressants and promising evidence for venlafaxine [34]. Medication may be particularly useful as psychological services in some areas are limited and following appropriate assessment the prescription of an antidepressant is relatively straightforward. A simple principle in the treatment of PTSD is 'sooner rather than later' to limit chronicity, and also to reduce the risk of the development of maladaptive coping mechanisms such as alcohol or substance misuse [34].

Psychological treatment approaches include prolonged exposure and cognitive restructuring [35] and eye movement desensitisation and reprocessing (EMDR) [36]. EMDR is a structured, multicomponent treatment package, which involves having the patient conjure up images of the traumatic event, its related thoughts and emotions, whilst engaging in bilateral stimulation in the form of saccadic eye movements, bilateral hand taps or bilateral auditory tones. Exposure in EMDR comes in short doses and incorporates a cognitive therapy component.

The prescription of a non-benzodiazepine sleeping tablet (such as zolpidem or zopiclone) after four consecutive nights of sleep disturbance is recommended. If after four weeks the patients' distress continues, a selective serotonin reuptake inhibitor (SSRI) should be prescribed (or earlier if the symptoms are particularly severe and they exhibit a number of risk factors). Patients should be informed that a trial of SSRI for PTSD will take 3 months and they will need to remain on the drug for a minimum of 6 months and up to 12–15 months for more severe or chronic PTSD. Adherence will be enhanced if they know that those showing some response at 3 months will continue to have additional benefits by 15 months [35].

Whilst the intensive care specialist can initiate first-line treatment, referral to a mental health specialist may be needed. Early referral should be considered when the PTSD is severe or there are worrying features, such as suicidal thoughts, or comorbid conditions, such as depression or substance misuse. Local availability of mental health services will vary and in some areas it may need to be provided in the private sector.

Conclusion

Over the last 20 years, the physical care of trauma victims and the critically ill has tended to advance more significantly than the psychiatric and psychological care. However, the psychological care should not be seen as less important. There is compelling evidence that traumatic experience triggers a psychological response, and for some patients a post-traumatic reaction such as PTSD may follow. Recent research has expanded knowledge about risk factors and it is now clear that whilst the stressor plays a key role, other factors relating to the trauma, the patient and the environment influence the development and persistence of post-traumatic psychomorbidity. Results are not consistent across trauma populations, and it is neither possible nor appropriate to create an overall vulnerability model for PTSD and related disorders. It is imperative therefore to identify risk factors for critical care patients. It should also be remembered that PTSD is not a normal adaptation to severe stress, nor is it an inevitable response to stress. If it does develop, many individuals will recover quickly from PTSD and if treatment is necessary, there is increasing empirical evidence for a variety of psychological and pharmacological treatments [34]. Predicting those at risk of post-trauma psychological disorders allows the early targeting of treatment.

References

1. American Psychiatric Association. *Diagnostic and Statistical Manual of Mental Disorders*, 4th Edn. Washington, DC: American Psychiatric Association, 1994.
2. World Health Organization. *The International Classification of Mental and Behavioural Disorders*, 10th Edn. Geneva: World Health Organization, 1992.

3. Mayou R, Bryant B. Outcome in consecutive emergency department attenders following road traffic accident. *B J Psychiatry* 2001;**179**:528–34.
4. Ballenger JC, Davidson JRT, Lecrubier Y, *et al*. Consensus Statement on Posttraumatic Stress Disorder from the International Consensus Group on Depression and Anxiety. *J Clin Psychiatry* 2000;**61**:S60–S66.
5. Kessler RC. Post-traumatic stress disorder: the burden to the individual and to society. *J Clin Psychiatry,* 2000;**61**:S4–S12.
6. Kulka RA, Schlenger WE, Fairbank JA, *et al*. *Trauma and the Vietnam War Generation: Report of Findings from the National Vietnam Veterans Readjustment Study.* New York: Brunner/Mazel, 1990.
7. O'Brien LS, Hughes SJ. Symptoms of post-traumatic stress disorder in Falklands veterans five years after the conflict. *B J Psychiatry* 1991;**159**:135–41.
8. Loughrey GC, Curren PS, Bell P. Posttraumatic stress disorder and civil violence in Northern Ireland. In: Wilson JP, Raphael B, eds. *International Handbook of Traumatic Stress Syndromes.* New York: Plenum Press, 1993, pp. 461–70.
9. Green BL, Lindy JD, Grace MC, *et al*. Buffalo Creek survivors in the second decade: stability of stress symptoms. *Am J Orthopsychiatry* 1990;**60**:43–54.
10. Kilpatrick DG, Resnick HS. Post-traumatic stress disorder associated with exposure to criminal victimization in clinical and community populations. In: Davidson JRT, Foa EB, eds. *Posttraumatic Stress Disorder: DSM-IV and beyond.* Washington, DC: American Psychiatric Press, 1992, pp. 113–43.
11. Hull AM, Lowe T, Devlin M, Finlay P, Stewart M. Psychological sequelae after maxillofacial trauma: a preliminary study. *Br J Oral Maxillofac Surg* 2003;**41**:317–22.
12. Cuthbertson BH, Hull AM, Strachan M, Scott J. Post-traumatic psychopathology after critical illness requiring general intensive care. *Intens Care Med* 2004;**30**:450–5.
13. Jones C, Griffiths RD, Humphris G, Skirrow PM. Memory, delusions, and the development of acute posttraumatic stress disorder-related symptoms after intensive care. *Crit Care Med* 2001;**29**:573–80.
14. Schelling G, Stoll C, Haller M, *et al*. Health-related quality of life and post-traumatic stress disorder in survivors of the acute respiratory distress syndrome. *Crit Care Med* 1998;**26**:651–9.
15. Scragg P, Jones A, Fauvel N. Psychological problems following ICU treatment. *Anaesthesia* 2001;**56**:9–14.
16. Yu BH, Dimsdale JE. Posttraumatic stress disorder in patients with burn injuries. *J Burn Care Rehabil* 1999;**20**:426–33.
17. Michaels AJ, Michaels CE, Zimmerman MA, *et al*. Post-traumatic stress disorder in injured adults: aetiology by path analysis. *J Trauma* 1999;**47**:867–73.
18. Stoll C, Schelling G, Goetz AE, *et al*. Health-related quality of life and post-traumatic stress disorder in patients after cardiac surgery and intensive care treatment. *J Thorac Cardiovasc Surg* 2000;**120**:505–12.
19. March JS. What constitutes a stressor? The "Criterion A" issue. In: Davidson JRT, Foa EB, eds. *Post-traumatic Stress Disorder: DSM-IV and Beyond.* Washington, DC: American Psychiatric Press, 1993, pp. 37–54.
20. Green BL. Psychosocial research in traumatic stress. *J Trauma Stress* 1994;**7**:341–62.
21. Klein S, Alexander DA, Hutchinson JD, *et al*. The Aberdeen Trauma Screening Index: an instrument to predict post-accident psychopathology. *Psychol Med* 2002;**32**:863–71.
22. Brewin CR, Andrews B, Valentine JD. Meta-analysis of risk factors for post-traumatic stress disorder in trauma-exposed adults. *J Consult Clin Psychol* 2000;**68**:748–66.

23. Gilbertson MW, Shenton ME, Ciszewski A, *et al.* Smaller hippocampal volume predicts pathologic vulnerability to psychological trauma. *Nat Neurosci* 2002;5:1242–7.
24. Hull AM. A review of neuroimaging findings in post-traumatic stress disorder. *B J Psychiatry* 2002;**181**:102–10.
25. Yehuda R, Schmeidler J, Wainberg M, *et al.* Increased vulnerability to post-traumatic stress disorder in adult offspring of Holocaust survivors. *Am J Psychiatry* 1998;**155**:1163–72.
26. Yehuda R. Biology of posttraumatic stress disorder. *J Clin Psychiatry* 2000; **61**:14–21.
27. McFarlane AC. Posttraumatic stress disorder: a model of the longitudinal course and the role of risk factors. *J Clin Psychiatry* 2000;**61**:15–23.
28. McFarlane AC, Atchison M, Yehuda R. The acute stress response following motor vehicle accidents and its relation to PTSD. *Ann N Y Acad Sci* 1997;**821**:437–41.
29. Delahunty DL, Raimonde AJ, Spoonster E. Initial post-traumatic urinary cortisol levels predict subsequent PTSD symptoms in motor vehicle accident victims. *Biol Psychiatry* 2000;**48**:940–7.
30. Resnick HS, Yehuda R, Pitman RK, *et al.* Effect of previous trauma on acute plasma cortisol level following rape. *Am J Psychiatry* 1995;**152**:1675–7.
31. Yehuda R. Post-traumatic stress disorder. *N Engl J Med* 2002;**346**:108–14.
32. Hull AM, Alexander DA, Klein S. A long-term follow-up study of survivors of the Piper Alpha Oil Platform Disaster. *B J Psychiatry* 2002;**181**:435–40.
33. Davidson JRT, Hughes D, Blazer DG, George LK. Post-traumatic stress disorder in the community: an epidemiological study. *Psychol Med* 1991;**21**:713–21.
34. Hull AM. Primary care management of post-traumatic stress disorder. *Prescriber* 2004;**15**:40–8.
35. Marks I, Lovell K, Noshirvani H, Livanou M, Thrasher S. Treatment of posttraumatic stress disorder by exposure and/or cognitive restructuring: a controlled study. *Arch Gen Psychiatry* 1998;**55**:317–25.
36. Shapiro F. Eye movement desensitization and reprocessing (EMDR): evaluation of controlled PTSD research. *J Behav Ther Exp Psychiatry* 1996; **27**:209–18.

3: Intensive care unit delirium, patients' perspective and clinical signs

ANETTH GRANBERG AXÈLL

Introduction

It is a myth that critically ill patients do not remember their intensive care stay. There are patients who remember nothing at all, but most patients can recall the time immediately following extubation and the following days with fragmentary memories (i.e. a jigsaw-puzzle memory). Patients describe 'events in sequences', particular objects, individual nurses, nursing actions and important emotional experiences. They are unable, for example, to describe their immediate surroundings or sometimes the time sequence of events. However, patients can remember in detail and describe their so-called 'unreal experiences' as a narrative story with a beginning, a middle and an end [1].

During the 1950s special units for monitoring and intensive therapy were developed. Soon staff became aware of major psychological and psychiatric disturbances among critically ill patients. These mental disturbances were given different names and various concepts were offered as explanations. The concept of intensive care unit syndrome (ICU syndrome) was first used by McKegney [2]. He established that patients' adaptation to stress seemed to have implications for outcome and indirectly for the development of ICU syndrome. During the 1990s the concept of ICU delirium was more widely recognised.

Lipowski [3] defined delirium as a mental disorder, which is characterised by acute onset, altered level of consciousness, fluctuating course and disturbances in orientation, memory, thought and behaviour. Kuch [4] concluded that the development of ICU delirium depended on a complex interaction of many factors. These include patients' previous psychological status, the psychological trauma inflicted by the illness, the environmental stressors inherent in ICU, and organic factors affecting the function of the central nervous system. The contributions of these four factors can vary considerably between patients as can the severity and type of resulting psychological disturbance.

Studies of ICU delirium have mainly described the objective symptoms and signs from the health care professional's perspective. Few studies are based on the patients' perspective of their experiences on ICU. One of the principal duties of the staff is to make patients feel safe, secure and comfortable. Another is to minimise suffering. It is therefore important to increase knowledge of ICU delirium so that care can be tailored to prevent the development of delirium or to limit its impact.

The aim of this chapter is to describe and explore ICU delirium from the patients' perspective and to investigate the clinical signs and demographic data associated with ICU delirium in patients mechanically ventilated for longer than 36 h [1,5,6,7].

Methods and patients

A variety of methodological approaches were used to explore patients' experiences. At Lund University, 31 general ICU patients (20 males, 11 females) were enrolled. These patients were mechanically ventilated for more than 36 h. Records were made during mechanical ventilation, the weaning process and the days following extubation [5].

Of these 31 patients, 19 were interviewed twice. The first interview usually took place on the recovery ward, between 6 and 10 days after ICU discharge. The second interview took place 4–8 weeks later usually in the patients' homes. The concept of an unreal experience was used when asking about their confusional states. In all, the interviews lasted for 2–5 h for each participant [6,7].

Findings

The findings cover a lot of themes and subjects and only a few will be presented here. A hermeneutical (i.e. concerning interpretation) approach was chosen as the overall principle in the analysis [5,6,7].

The chaos experienced when becoming critically ill or seriously injured

Patients' own reports suggest that the basis for developing ICU delirium is their experiences of pain, fear, loss of control, vulnerability, emptiness, passivity and altered body awareness. Some of these unpleasant experiences appear before their ICU admission. Some patients say that they were 'crazy or mad' or had a 'nervous breakdown' due to the pain or illness before their

ICU admission. This may start a series of frightening experiences, which are related to threats to existence, the struggle for survival and the risk of death as their bodies seem to have failed to function properly.

The 'waking up' period

The time taken for patients to become fully awake after sedation has worn off or been withdrawn differed from a couple of hours to several days. Most patients seemed to be calmed by the presence of relatives and a nurse and the explanations offered. However, some patients displayed violent unco-ordinated movements during weaning, as if they were in some sort of fury because they could not be understood. Some even tried to pull out their tubes and get out of bed. These patients showed signs of anxiety, panic, and even antipathy and hatred towards the staff.

The presence of their relatives was one of their first real memories. The relatives represented normality and offered a lifeline patient's of reality for the patient. This relationship seemed to confirm the patient's existence, bringing order to chaos and providing security.

Another initial memory was extubation itself. Half of the 19 patients remembered how it was carried out, the sound of the ventilator and a sore throat. Their memories of extubation were sometimes associated with unreal experiences and fear. Extubation also started a struggle for survival. The fear of not being able to breathe, being suffocated, created feelings of dying, a threat to life that could persist for several days.

Patients' sensitivity and vulnerability

Patients' first feelings upon waking are of emptiness of both mind and body 'as if the body were sailing and alien'. The patients do not know where they are, what has happened, the time of day or even which day it is. Their minds are wide open and they feel defenceless and believe that anything could happen. All kinds of feelings are experienced. These feelings could be contradictory (i.e. both hope and despair, security and insecurity, fear and safety). Some patients said that they felt completely empty, void of any thoughts or feelings and that they could not talk normally. Patients also report that they had to make an effort to regain control over their strangely empty bodies.

Experiences of being unable to sleep

Upon waking up, several patients reported that they felt totally exhausted (e.g. 'I felt that I had been walking for ten miles'). In spite of this, it was often impossible for them to sleep, even if they were no longer connected to the ventilator. 'I could not sleep, although I wanted to, I just couldn't relax.' It seems that in order to be able to sleep, the patient must first be able to relax. A common statement was that 'it was impossible to sleep due to all the noise'. Another patient said she was afraid to sleep, as she was concerned about waking up intubated again, and she was afraid that if she fell asleep she would never wake up again.

Patients frequently reported unreal experiences during the night and this made them scared of falling asleep. Sleep often started with a series of unreal experiences that were often experienced as horrific and triggered patients' fear of becoming mad. Falling asleep is thus associated with fear and the recall of unreal experiences.

During the study, 2–6 h following extubation some of the patients seemed to be able to rest peacefully, while others, even if they seemed tired or completely exhausted, could not rest at all. Some patients seemed quite 'normal' in their behaviour until they attempted to rest; they fell asleep for a few minutes and then suddenly became anxious, restless, plucking at the sheets and mumbling. The patients' ability to rest peacefully appears to be an important predictor of ICU delirium in that many delirious patients are also sleep-deprived.

Experiences of time and day

Some patients described how they fought to regain perception of time. This struggle was often associated with unreal experiences. Their fight to regain control over time could become a nightmare as, according to the patients' perception, time stood completely still. Patients also report difficulties in distinguishing night from day, and say that several days and nights were totally missing from their memory. They talked in terms of 'missing days' and that this lost time felt like a violation of their personal space and integrity.

Patients' experiences of thoughts, speech, language and communication

Several patients said that their speech did not function normally. They could not make themselves understood and therefore were unable to communicate and share experiences or feelings with others. When they awoke connected to peculiar machines and apparatus, they felt like aliens or strangers being tied down in their beds. Patients recall that their voices did not obey them and it was impossible to think properly, so the words used were not the words they wanted to say. They say that it felt as if there were no connection between their brain and their mouth.

A few patients said that they felt relatively well and that their speech functioned normally. One patient describes that he felt calm and satisfied, and was able to think quite clearly and even ask some questions. But later when resting, he said he was awoken by a loud noise and felt frightened. Suddenly, he did not know where he was or what had happened. He tried to tell the nurse about this but he could not find the right words as his speech was slurred and he said the wrong things. This fluctuating ability to communicate and control body movements seems to be connected with fear and anxiety. However, patients may be able to conceal their anxiety and confusion.

Patients' descriptions of their unreal experience

Several patients spontaneously described unreal experiences of different kinds. They usually used special phrases when describing these, such as dreams, nightmares, stupid fantasies, changes of perspective, crazy dreams, illusions or dreamlike experiences. Only one patient used the concept of hallucination; sometimes, individual phrases or metaphors were used. The concept of unreal experiences is most appropriate here, as the patient somehow knows that these experiences are unreal but are nonetheless very vivid. When these unreal experiences occurred, patients were usually fully awake with their eyes open. 'It was as if it were real, as if it were really happening.'

Unreal experiences also concerned escaping from ICU and returning home. One patient said that he felt like two persons, where one of them had been given his clothes and returned home, while the other one was forced to stay at a cheap hotel (i.e. the hospital). Another type of unreal experience was changes in the appearance and perspective of their rooms. One patient said: 'it happened right in front of my eyes.' Patients considered themselves to be fully awake and these changes were reality at that time. One such example was that the floor around the bed turned into a 2 m deep trench. The patient described the struggle with himself – one part wanting to get up and see if there really was a trench around his bed, while the other told him to stay in bed. Each time the patient woke up, he experienced this trench around his bed. This continued for about 1 day.

The variety and extent of ICU delirium

Based on the observations and the patients' descriptions of acute confusion, dysfunctional speech and thought and their unreal experiences, they were classified into three groups: severe delirium, moderate delirium and mild delirium [5,6,7].

Severe delirium

Patients with severe delirium reported that their unreal experiences, which could last for several days, were already present when they regained consciousness. In addition, these patients describe disorientation, difficulties in speaking and sleeping, together with severe chaotic feelings and bizarre experiences. They usually felt an overwhelming fear that they were out of control and fighting for survival. They struggled to regain control of their own body and wanted to escape from everything. Emotionally, they fluctuated between feelings of security and insecurity, fear and hope. Irritation, anger and aggression dominated their feelings, which were chaotic and uncontrollable.

The notes from the observations indicated that patients with severe delirium made violent uncoordinated movements, as if they were in some sort of fury. In the hours after extubation and/or in the evening, most of them mumbled to themselves and/or talked continuously. These patients showed signs of anxiety, panic and antipathy or hatred towards the staff. All of them repeatedly tried to get out of bed and the nurses had severe difficulty in convincing them that they had to stay in bed because of their condition. They had great sleeping difficulties.

Moderate delirium

Patients with moderate delirium reported a few unreal experiences, which often returned for a couple of hours, usually occurring or developing during the days following extubation. These patients felt emotionally vulnerable, but as a rule, they believed that they were in control of themselves and could understand and remember information. Many in this group reported feelings of trust and confidence in the nurses. However, they did experience fear and uneasiness all the time, and anything, even apparently small and unimportant events, could trigger unreal experiences. When these patients were observed, they appeared to be fully awake 1 or 2 h after withdrawal of the sedative drugs. Patients seemed to be calmed by their relatives and the nurses' presence and explanations. They communicated normally with the nurses and were curious about the other patients. However, they could suddenly change from being able to communicate adequately to mumbling and becoming incoherent. This fluctuating level in communication and control of their body movements seemed connected with fear and anxiety.

Mild delirium

The group of patients with mild delirium described that they had only experienced disturbed day and time perception, with some having difficulty regaining their normal day perception. A few experienced emotional chaos and reported a mild disorientation. These patients said that it was very trying, as they thought someone or something had 'stolen their time'. They could not describe or remember any unreal experiences, dreams or nightmares. These patients were partly disoriented, could talk properly and did not report any unreal experiences or display any signs of mumbling speech or restlessness. They were able to rest and sleep without any difficulty.

Conclusion

The concept of ICU delirium implies a cause-and-effect relationship with the medical condition, the psychological trauma and the critical care environment. Patients described a state of chaos, which generally started when they fell ill or were injured. This seems to originate in the feeling that life is threatened because the body is no longer functioning properly and in the sense of loss of control of body, mind and environment. The immediate and most profound feeling in this chaos is fear, which may become transformed into a persistent inner tension or prolonged fear. However, in conjunction with this fear, some patients describe an underlying hope related to life, which could be strengthened by relatives and other staff. The loss of control and the chaos described by the patients may well be fundamental factors behind the development of ICU delirium. Clinical signs and patients' verbal expressions must be regarded as a coherent whole. This assumes, however, that we believe that patients' behaviour is intentional and has a meaning and that it conveys some kind of message that can be interpreted or may be understood. ICU delirium can be seen as a uniquely developed pattern for each patient.

References

1. Granberg AA. The intensive care unit syndrome/delirium, patients' perspective and clinical signs. Lund University: Doctoral dissertation, 2001, ISBN 91-628-4624-8.
2. McKegney FP. The intensive care syndrome: the definition, treatment and prevention of a new "disease of medical progress". *Connect Med* 1966;**30**:633.
3. Lipowski ZJ. *Delirium: Acute Confusional States.* Oxford: Oxford University Press, 1990.
4. Kuch K. Anxiety disorders and the ICU. *Clin Intens Care* 1990;**1**:7–11.
5. Granberg AA, Bergbom-Engberg I, Lundberg D. Clinical signs of ICU syndrome/delirium: an observational study. *Intens Crit Care Nurs* 2001;**17**:72–93.
6. Granberg AA, Bergbom-Engberg I, Lundberg D. Patients' experience of being critically ill or severely injured and cared for in an intensive care unit in relation to the ICU syndrome. Part I. *Intensive Crit Care Nurs* 1998;**14**:294–307.
7. Granberg AA, Bergbom-Engberg I, Lundberg D. Acute confusion and unreal experiences in intensive care patients in relation to the ICU syndrome. Part II. *Intens Crit Care Nurs* 1999;**15**:19–33.

Further reading

Granberg AA, Bergbom-Engberg I, Lundberg D. Intensive care syndrome: a literature review. *Intens Crit Care Nurs* 1996;**12**:173–82.

Granberg AA, Malmros C, Bergbom-Engberg I, Lundberg D. Intensive care unit syndrome/delirium is associated with anemia, drug therapy and duration of ventilation treatment. *Acta Anaesthesiol Scand* 2002;**46**:726–31.

4: Delirium and confusion: more than ICU syndrome

RICHARD D GRIFFITHS, CHRISTINA JONES

Introduction

The rapid growth and technical developments of intensive care have saved patients from life-threatening conditions associated with profound metabolic and inflammatory disturbances that 50 years ago would have been fatal. Mechanical ventilation and other aspects of intensive care involve the high-dose use of sedatives and analgesics for prolonged periods. Myriad behavioural and psychiatric changes have been observed that have been termed 'ICU syndrome' or 'ICU psychosis' as the collective aetiology was considered uniquely related to the intensive care unit (ICU). However, describing causation to an environmental exposure is misguided, serving little clinical purpose and offering no management guidance. Furthermore, as we have studied the outcome and problems of patients after intensive care, many of the simplistic assumptions appear incorrect and new evidence is challenging what is considered best for our patients. We now recognise that it is the patients who suffer delirium while the staff are 'confused' as to what is going on and what is best for the patients.

Delirium is a medical condition

Delirium is characterised by an acutely changing or fluctuating mental status, inattention, disorganised thinking, and altered consciousness that may or may not be accompanied by agitation. Hallucinations may also be associated with delirium. While the behavioural anomaly of aggressiveness is easy to notice, that of passivity may be less apparent. One of the criteria in the *Diagnostic and Statistical Manual of Mental Disorders*, 4th edition (DSM-IV) of the American Psychiatric Association [1] for the diagnosis of delirium includes evidence of effects of a general medical condition, medicine or substance intoxication or withdrawal (Box 4.1). It is not surprising therefore that the incidence of delirium is dependent on the patient population and ranges from 0–40% post-operatively [2] to 19–80% [3] or over 80% [4]

within intensive care. Furthermore, the presence and duration of delirium is a strong predictor of length of hospital stay after correcting for severity of illness, age and days of sedative use. Not surprisingly the most frequent risk factor within ICU is benzodiazepine or narcotic use, while a history of smoking, alcohol and hypertension are predisposing factors (Table 4.1).

Box 4.1 The criteria for the diagnosis of delirium cited in the American Psychiatric Association's *Diagnostic and Statistical Manual of Mental Disorders* **[1]**

A. Disturbance of consciousness (i.e. reduced clarity of awareness of the environment) with reduced ability to focus, sustain, or shift attention.

B. A change in cognition (such as memory deficit, disorientation, language disturbance) or the development of a perceptual disturbance that is not better accounted for by a pre-existing, established, or evolving dementia.

C. The disturbance develops over a short period of time (usually hours to days) and tends to fluctuate during the course of the day.

D. There is evidence from the history, physical examination, or laboratory findings that the disturbance is caused directly by one of the following:

   i. physiological consequences of a general medical condition

   ii. result of medication use or substance intoxication

   iii. result of a withdrawal syndrome

   iv. result of more than one of the above aetiologies

Table 4.1 Risk factors for delirium in ICU [3]

Variable on multivariate analysis	Odds ratio	95% CI
Prior hypertension	2.6	1.14–5.72
Smoking history	2.2	0.94–4.94
Bilirubin abnormal	1.2	1.03–1.40
Use of epidural analgesia	3.5	1.20–10.3
Morphine analgesia use	9.2	2.17–39.0

Odds ratio: the odds that a patient with delirium has been exposed to a variable (e.g. the odds that a patient becomes delirious after receiving morphine as an analgesic are 9.2 times greater than a patient who did not receive morphine).
CI: confidence interval.

Intensive care patients are not a simple cross section of society but rather a select population with a higher incidence of diseases related to smoking and excess alcohol consumption.

The Confusion Assessment Method for the ICU (CAM-ICU) [5] is a validated, practical and reliable assessment tool to diagnose delirium in ICU (Box 4.2). It is recommended for routine use by the guidelines for sedation of the American Society of Critical Care Medicine [6]. The first part of the CAM-ICU looks for evidence of an acute change and fluctuating mental status in the past 24 h. As patients with delirium find it difficult to sustain attention, the second part of the CAM-ICU uses a simple attention-screening test, which is completely non-verbal and only requires that the patient can squeeze the examiner's hand or nod his or her head. The third

---

Box 4.2 The Confusion Assessment Method for the Intensive Care Unit (CAM-ICU) [5]

Delirium is diagnosed when both Features 1 and 2 are present, along with either Feature 3 or Feature 4.

Feature 1. Acute onset of mental status changes or fluctuating course

- Is there evidence of an acute change in mental status from the baseline?
- Did the (abnormal) behaviour fluctuate during the past 24 h, that is, tend to come and go or increase and decrease in severity?

Sources of information: Serial Glasgow Coma Scale or sedation score ratings over 24 h as well as readily available input from the patient's bedside critical care nurse or family.

Feature 2. Inattention

- Did the patient have difficulty focusing attention?
- Is there a reduced ability to maintain and shift attention?

Sources of information: Attention-screening examinations by using either picture recognition or a random letter test. Neither of these tests requires verbal response, and so they are ideally suited for mechanically ventilated patients.

Feature 3. Disorganised thinking

- Was the patient's thinking disorganised or incoherent, such as rambling or irrelevant conversation, unclear or illogical flow of ideas, or unpredictable switching from subject to subject?

Continued on Page 31

- Was the patient able to follow questions and commands throughout the assessment?

  1. "Are you having any unclear thoughts?"
  2. "Hold up this many fingers." (examiner holds two fingers in front of the patient)
  3. "Now, do the same thing with the other hand." (not repeating the number of fingers)

Feature 4. Altered level of consciousness (i.e. any level of consciousness other than alert)

- Alert – normal, spontaneously fully aware of environment and interacts appropriately
- Vigilant – hyperalert
- Lethargic – drowsy but easily aroused, unaware of some elements in the environment, or not spontaneously interacting appropriately with the interviewer; becomes fully aware and appropriately interactive when prodded minimally
- Stupor – difficult to arouse, unaware of some or all elements in the environment, or not spontaneously interacting with the interviewer; becomes incompletely aware and inappropriately interactive when prodded strongly
- Coma – unarousable, unaware of all elements in the environment, with no spontaneous interaction or awareness of the interviewer, so that the interview is difficult or impossible even with maximal prodding

criterion for delirium is disorganised thinking. If a patient is still intubated, there is a set of questions to which he or she can respond non-verbally (e.g. will a stone float on water?). The fourth and final part of the test looks for any evidence of altered level of consciousness (e.g. reduced Glasgow Coma Score). The diagnosis of delirium using the CAM-ICU requires the first two criteria to be met in conjunction with either the third or fourth.

The fundamental causes of delirium are pathophysiological factors rather than the many theoretical causes related to sleep disturbances, psychological factors and the 'special' influence of the ICU environment. Delirium is an important diagnosis that assists medical management and symptom control [7]. The most common medical causes of delirium are metabolic disturbances, electrolyte imbalances, withdrawal syndromes, acute infections (intracranial and systemic) and central nervous system disorders (seizures, space-occupying lesions, vascular disorders). Medicine intoxication and withdrawal are compounded by altered pharmacokinetics associated with increasing age and multiple organ dysfunction. Pre-existing cognitive decline in the elderly will compound delirium management.

Encephalopathy is common in ICU

Only recently have we started to appreciate the severity and extent of cerebral pathology occurring in critically ill patients, especially those with severe sepsis and multiple organ failure. Sensory evoked potentials (SEPs) have quantified cerebral function in early sepsis. In a study of 68 patients with severe sepsis, 84% of patients showed severity of illness-related impairment in cortical SEPs within the first 48 h [8]. Such septic encephalopathy may be more frequent than is generally assumed. More recently from France, a detailed histological study of brain tissue has compared the changes in patients dying early from septic shock with two control groups (patients dying from non-septic shock or suddenly from overwhelming extracranial injury). Ischaemic and apoptotic (programmed cell death) changes were extensive and were greater in patients with septic and non-septic shock compared to those dying suddenly. Ischaemic changes were most marked in the septic shock patients and were found in the lenticular nuclei, amygdala and autonomic nuclei. Even more striking, however, was the significantly increased neuronal apoptosis in the amygdala, supraoptic, paraventricular and medullary autonomic nuclei of patients dying of septic shock compared with either control group. There was a good correlation with markers of inducible nitric oxide synthase expression suggesting a relationship to severity of vascular inflammation, while there was less relationship with the duration or severity of hypotension. These pathological changes may relate to neurotransmitter alterations (cholinergic, serotonergic, dopaminergic or gamma-aminobutyric acid) that are all implicated in the pathophysiology of delirium [9] (Figure 4.1). Widespread disruption including damage to the amygdala, the centre involved in the emotional overtones of memory, may account for the disturbed memory and amnesia in critical illness, possibly explaining the recall of life-threatening delusions despite amnesia of ICU [10].

ICU psychosis has no strong scientific basis for being unique to ICU

The direct causal effect of sleep disturbance and deprivation in ICU syndrome is weak. Normal volunteers develop perceptual anomalies with sleep deprivation but these bear little relationship to distressing delusions [11].

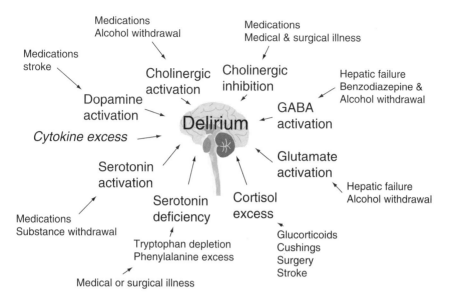

Figure 4.1 The possible causes and pathophysiology of delirium.

Many studies have shown correlation between severity of illness and sleep disturbance. Therefore it is possible that the physical illness itself is responsible and not necessarily the sleep disturbance. In a review of 80 studies of post-operative delirious patients, lack of sleep was not a predisposing factor [2]. Similarly, disturbances of the circadian rhythm assessed by temperature nadir have failed to show a relationship with ICU psychosis [12]. However, another study suggested there was a relationship with low melatonin secretion after thoracic surgery [13]. Melatonin secretion measured by the urinary metabolite 6-sulphatoxymelatonin was elevated in patients with sepsis versus non-septic controls. This led to an impaired circadian rhythm in septic patients whereas in the non-septic patients periodicity was still present [14].

Many of the proposed theories trying to explain ICU psychosis include an array of contradictory factors that appear to ignore the underlying medical pathology and fail to provide sufficient evidence of mechanisms to explain the delirium. Although the prior psychological state and experience may influence the delirium, there is no personality profile that can predict post-operative delirium [15] and the environmental stressors cannot explain problems in patients who have complete amnesia for ICU. The predisposing factors for delirium in ICU remain closely associated with markers of the underlying illness such as anaemia, metabolic acidosis, uraemia, jaundice, and use of common ICU drugs including dopamine and duration of ventilation [4,16,17,18].

The psychological challenges of delirium in ICU

Because delirium is so frequent in ICU, incorrectly diagnosing acute anxiety in an agitated patient or acute depression in a passive patient should be avoided. Using intensive care follow-up, it is possible to identify a number of key points to help patient management. These include:

(a) Patients have different kinds of hallucinations and delusions. While some may be pleasant and transitory, others are unpleasant delusional experiences that may be held as firm beliefs. The most strongly held beliefs tend to be persecutory and even life-threatening [19].

(b) The behaviour of patients may be strongly influenced by their present delusion but this may not be apparent to their carers. For instance, a patient showing profound compliance and no obvious outward distress had developed Capgas Syndrome, a disorder of face recognition leading to a delusional belief that everyone but she had been replaced by aliens. She reasoned that if she failed to comply with the nurses she would be replaced [20].

(c) Patients have difficulty in remembering real events and can misinterpret events if sufficiently aware [10]. Accurately remembering real events enables patients to orientate themselves and recognise hallucinations or delusional experiences. Furthermore, despite the many unpleasant aspects of ICU, the most important experience for such patients is that someone is looking after them, providing security and safety.

(d) The delusion can be influenced by events or experiences immediately before the severe illness. For instance, the incidence of delusions containing military themes increased during intense media coverage of a recent war and also occurred uniquely in patients who would have been young adults during World War II [21].

(e) Patients who are amnesic of any real ICU event may have the entire experience replaced by a strongly held delusional belief. If this is persecutory and in particular life-threatening, it can predispose to developing the post-traumatic stress disorder (PTSD) [22]. The combination of a vivid life-threatening experience and the loss of personal safety due to amnesia of ICU are key components.

Within intensive care, excluding delirium is an important first step and involves a systematic medical approach with formal testing using the CAM-ICU. Even with delirium excluded, the inability of patients to vocalise makes establishing alternative diagnoses difficult. Precipitous and indiscriminate use of anxiolytics and antidepressants should be avoided.

Implication for management in ICU

Depression or PTSD after discharge from ICU is now well recognised (see Chapters 2 and 5). PTSD has been associated with a number of stressors usually perceived as unpleasant ICU experiences. Our own research shows that patients who have delusional experiences in association with amnesia for ICU develop acute stress reactions and tend to go on to develop more frequent PTSD-related symptoms [22]. In contrast, patients who have delusional experiences in association with some recall of ICU have a significantly lower incidence of PTSD, which is similar to that of patients without delusions. In critically ill patients, the stressor is the life-threatening delusional experience when the patient is amnesic of the surroundings and devoid of the perception of support and safety. Such memories are often intrusive and may be more firmly retained than those of actual experiences and so more available to recall. The association of stress reactions and delirium has been previously described [23]. In 34 delirious burns patients, 7 out of 25 survivors had severe psychological symptoms of either depression or PTSD [24]. Their delusions resulted in stronger and longer-lasting intrusive and fearful memories of their personal injury. The patients could generally recall their injury. This contrasted with the other survivors who had delusional experiences that were either pleasant or unrelated to personal injury. PTSD can follow an acute psychosis and the mechanism is believed to be due to the delusional experience rather than real events [25].

These observations have implications for how we manage patients on ICU. Avoiding delirium is clearly desirable but the nature of the diseases and of our patients makes this harder. If the actual ICU experience can partly protect against delusional related stress disorders, lighter sedation may be preferable for patients so that they are more aware of their surroundings, however unpleasant we may perceive them to be.

Implication for management after ICU

These observations also have implications for how we manage patients after ICU. As a means of gaining feedback on the critical care received by patients and their relatives, it has been suggested that the National Health Service (NHS) adopt methods used in other care settings. Despite lack of firm evidence, it is suggested that single 'discovery interviews' would fill this role and could be applied independent of formal follow-up services. The combination of highly distorted and delusional experiences of ICU and psychological distress after intensive care seriously questions the validity of this process [26]. A one-off discovery interview is similar to the debriefing undertaken to help individuals cope with traumatic events.

Unfortunately, research suggests that a single debriefing session may actually increase the risk of developing PTSD [27]. Without recognition and sufficient ongoing support of vulnerable individuals, such single interviews may increase the risk of PTSD for both patients and relatives. A recent meta-analysis of single-session debriefing after psychological trauma showed that it may impede recovery [28]. Ideally such debriefing interviews should be part of a multicomponent therapy that includes formal ICU follow-up and pathways for referral for further management. It is also fundamental that the validity of any information gained from patients be verified before care is altered based upon false recall arising from distorted perceptions or delusional experiences.

Many critical care patients have poor factual recall for both their admission to hospital and their intensive care stay, or their memories may be delusional (e.g. hospital staff trying to kill them) [10]. Such patients frequently express a desire to learn what really happened to them, and their relatives often have specific questions. It is therefore fundamental that staff interviewing patients after ICU have a comprehensive knowledge of the clinical care of the patients. In addition, a small proportion of patients remain convinced that their memories of staff trying to kill them are really what happened.

Conclusion

Rehabilitation following critical illness requires a clear understanding by the patient of what has occurred. Delirium and amnesia make this a challenge. Not only is there a duty of care by intensive care doctors to tell patients what has happened while they were under their care but there is also the need to offer explanations [29]. Our observations over almost 15 years of ICU follow-up confirm the benefit of rebuilding the autobiographical memory through careful discussion with patients and relatives by intensive care doctors or nurses [30], on the wards [31] and in clinics [32]. The added help of contemporaneously recorded diaries with pictures help patients come to terms with their illness and understand their rehabilitation [33] (see Chapter 8). Persistent or unrecognised psychological problems after intensive care are common. It is possible to enhance physical recovery, but in some patients psychological problems slow their recovery and require more specific therapy [34]. The term 'ICU syndrome' should not be used but rather 'delirium' used to describe the collective manifestations of organic brain disease in ICU that produces significant psychological problems.

References

1. American Psychiatric Association. *Diagnostic and Statistical Manual of Mental Disorders*, 4th Edn. Washington, DC: American Psychiatric Association, 1994, pp. 123–33.
2. Dyer CB, Ashton CM, Teasdale TA. Postoperative delirium: a review of 80 primary data-collection studies. *Arch Intern Med* 1995;**155**:461–5.
3. Dubois M-J, Bergeron N, Dumont M, Dial S, Skrobik Y. Delirium in an intensive care unit: a study of risk factors. *Intens Care Med* 2001;**27**:1297–1304.
4. Ely EW, Gautam S, Margolin R, *et al.* The impact of delirium in the intensive care unit on hospital length of stay. *Intens Care Med* 2001;**27**:1892–1900.
5. Ely EW, Margolin R, Francis J, *et al.* Evaluation of delirium in critically ill patients: validation of the confusion assessment method for the intensive care unit (CAM-ICU). *Crit Care Med* 2001;**29**:1370–9.
6. Jacobi J, Fraser GL, Coursin DB, *et al.* Clinical practice guidelines for the sustained use of sedatives and analgesics in the critically ill adult. *Crit Care Med* 2002;**30**:119–41.
7. McGuire BE, Basten CJ, Ryan CJ, Gallagher J. Intensive care unit syndrome: a dangerous misnomer. *Arch Intern Med* 2000;**160**:906–9.
8. Zauner C, Gendo A, Kramer L, *et al.* Impaired subcortical and cortical sensory evoked potential pathways in septic patients. *Crit Care Med* 2002;**30**:1136–9.
9. Flacker JM, Lipsitz LA. Neural mechanisms of delirium: current hypotheses and evolving concepts. *J Gerontol A Biol Sci Med Sci* 1999;**54A**:B239–46.
10. Jones C, Griffiths RD, Humphris G. Disturbed memory and amnesia related to intensive care. *Memory* 2000;**8**:79–94.
11. Morris GO, Williams HL, Lubin A. Misperception and disorientation during sleep deprivation. *Arch Gen Psychiatry* 1960;**2**:247–54.
12. Nuttall GA, Kumar M, Murray MJ. No difference exists in the alteration of circadian rhythm between patients with and without intensive care unit psychosis. *Crit Care Med* 1998;**26**:1351–5.
13. Myazaki T, Kuwano H, Kato H, *et al.* Correlation between serum melatonin circadian rhythm and intensive care unit psychosis after thoracic esophagectomy. *Surgery* 2003;**133**:662–8.
14. Mundigler G, Delle-Karth G, Koreny M, *et al.* Impaired circadian rhythm of melatonin secretion in sedated critically ill patients with severe sepsis. *Crit Care Med* 2002;**30**:536–40.
15. Dubin MD, Field HL, Gastfried BS. Postcardiotomy delirium: a review. *J Thorac Cardiovasc Surg* 1979;**77**:586–94.
16. Granberg AA, Malmros C, Bergbom-Engberg I, Lundberg D. Intensive care unit syndrome/delirium is associated with anaemia, drug therapy and duration of ventilation. *Acta Anaesthesiol Scand* 2002;**46**:726–31.
17. Aldemir M, Ozen S, Kara IH, Sir A, Bac B. Predisposing factors for delirium in the surgical intensive care unit. *Crit Care* 2001;**5**:265–70.
18. Sommer BR, Wise LC, Kraemer HC. Is dopamine administration possibly a risk factor for delirium? *Crit Care Med* 2002;**30**:1508–11.
19. Skirrow P. Delusional memories of ICU. In: Griffiths RD, Jones C, eds. *Intensive Care Aftercare*. Oxford: Butterworth-Heinemann. 2002, pp. 27–35.
20. Jones C, Griffiths RD, Humphris GM. A case of Capgras' delusion following critical illness. *Intens Care Med* 1999;**25**:183–4.
21. Skirrow P, Jones C, Griffiths RD, Kaney S. The impact of current media events on hallucinatory content: the experience of the intensive care unit (ICU) patient. *Br J Clin Psychol* 2002;**41**:87–91.

22. Jones C, Griffiths RD, Humphris G. Acute post-traumatic stress disorder: a new theory for its development after intensive care. *Crit Care Med* 2001;**29**:573–80.
23. Mackenzie TB, Popkin MK. Stress response syndrome occurring after delirium. *Am J Psychiatry* 1980;**137**:1433–5.
24. Blank K, Perry S. Relationship of psychological process during delirium to outcome. *Am J Pscyshiatry* 1984;**141**:843–7.
25. Shaw K, McFarlane AC, Bookless C, Air T. The aetiology of postpsychotic posttraumatic stress disorder following a psychotic episode. *J Trauma Stress* 2002;**15**:39–47.
26. Jones C, Griffiths RD, Waldmann C. Discovery interviews or mystery tours? *Care of the Crit Ill* 2003;**19**:103.
27. Bisson J, Jenkins P, Alexander J, Bannister C. A randomised controlled trial of psychological debriefing for victims of acute burn trauma. *Br J Psychiatry* 1997;**171**:78–81.
28. van Emmerik AAP, Kamphuis JH, Hulsbosch AM, Emmelkamp PMG. Single session debriefing after psychological trauma: a meta-analysis. *Lancet* 2002;**360**:766–71.
29. Griffiths RD, Jones C. Why is ICU follow-up needed? In: Griffiths RD, Jones C, eds. *Intensive Care Aftercare.* Oxford: Butterworth-Heinemann, 2002, pp. 1–4.
30. Jones C, Griffiths RD. Physical and psychological recovery. In: Griffiths RD, Jones C, eds. *Intensive Care Aftercare.* Oxford: Butterworth-Heinemann, 2002, pp. 53–65.
31. Carr K. Ward visits after intensive care discharge: why? In: Griffiths RD, Jones C, eds. *Intensive Care Aftercare.* Oxford: Butterworth-Heinemann, 2002, pp. 69–82.
32. Griffiths RD, Jones C. Recovery after intensive care: ABC of intensive care. *Br Med J* 1999;**319**:427–9.
33. Backman C. Patient diaries in ICU. In: Griffiths RD, Jones C, eds. *Intensive Care Aftercare.* Oxford: Butterworth-Heinemann, 2002, pp. 125–9.
34. Jones C, Skirrow P, Griffiths RD, *et al.* Rehabilitation after critical illness: a randomised, controlled trial. *Crit Care Med* 2003;**31**:2456–61.

5: Psychological stress in adult ICU patients and relatives

CHRISTINA JONES, RICHARD D GRIFFITHS

Introduction

Critical illness places severe physiological stress upon most organ systems within the body. It is now recognised that critical illness is associated with psychological stress in both patients and their relatives. Such psychological stress may well result from anatomical cerebral changes in patients while in relatives the unexpected, unfamiliar and frightening environment may contribute. Critical care practitioners need to be aware and recognise such psychological stress in their patients and relatives so that their treatment may be more complete.

Psychological stress in the intensive care unit – patients

The patient population in the intensive care unit (ICU) is mixed and varies considerably between units. Post-operative patients may experience a strong sense of security as they wake up if they were advised of, and prepared for, their admission [1]. Emergency patients' perception of their surroundings and comprehension of information will be clouded as they awake from sedation. As the effects of sedation and illness lessen, symptoms of anxiety and depression have been reported [2,3,4]. In serious illness, anxiety, panic attacks and depression are common [5]. Patients in ICU are emotionally and physically dependent on the staff looking after them. Provision of security, information, hope and emotional support is sufficient to help many patients cope. Psychotropic drugs should be avoided if possible as they may further cloud cognition. A recent study found that feeling vulnerable was reduced when patients were well informed, they received care that was personalised to their own needs and had a family member present [6].

Psychological stress in the intensive care unit – relatives

Families of critical care patients often experience enormous stress. A large multicentred study showed that 73% of family members and 84% of spouses reported symptoms of anxiety or depression while their relative was in ICU [7]. However, the support given to relatives by ICU nurses, in the form of information, advice and guidance, can ameliorate some anxiety [8]. Despite this, ICU experience is clearly traumatic and many relatives report feeling powerless and frightened. This experience may predispose ICU relatives to later psychological problems.

Psychological stress after critical care discharge

For patients and relatives, a major stressor is critical care discharge, particularly when this takes place at night. Regardless of preparation on ICU, the dramatic difference in the levels of care in critical care areas and the general wards is such that families frequently feel abandoned. Moving from ICU with its 1 : 1 nurse–patient ratio to a large general ward is a tremendous challenge for patients and their relatives. Warning patients and their families about this does not lessen its impact. A follow-up visit as soon as possible after discharge when the family are present allows any fears and worries to be discussed.

Anxiety and depression are common in patients and their families after discharge. For close family members, high levels of anxiety symptoms are predictive of developing the post-traumatic stress disorder (PTSD) [9]. One study involving 3655 patients reported problems with younger patients aged between 30 and 50 years, particularly with emotional behaviour, sleep and alertness [10]. A summary of recent studies of psychological problems in patients and relatives is given in Table 5.1. Survivors experience considerable levels of depression, anxiety, irritability and social isolation after discharge from hospital [11]. In addition, PTSD is more likely if patients can recall frightening delusional memories of ICU, such as nightmares, hallucinations and paranoid delusions. Where delusional memories are the sole recollections of ICU, the risk of developing PTSD is even higher [12]. In addition, there is a strong correlation between symptom levels in family members and patients [9]. This may be because the patient and relatives are unable to support each other.

Although physical recovery can be improved by the use of self-directed rehabilitation packages early in the convalescent phase, psychological recovery may not be as simple [8]. While depression may be improved, self-directed packages have less impact on anxiety and symptoms of PTSD. This is particularly so when patients report delusional memories, so emphasising the importance of recognising such patients and ensuring an appropriate referral for further treatment.

Table 5.1 Summary of several studies examining psychological recovery

Study	Subgroup	Patient numbers	Anxiety (%)	Depression (%)	PTSD (%)
Patients					
Jones *et al.* 1994 [11]	—	28	55.5	—	—
Koshy *et al.* 1997 [29]	—	50	—	—	15
Schelling *et al.* 1998 [30]	ARDS	80	—	—	27.5
Nelson *et al.* 2000 [31]	ARDS	24	43.5	—	25
Schnyder *et al.* 2001 [32]	Trauma	106	—	—	14
Scragg *et al.* 2001 [33]	—	80	47	47	15
Jones *et al.* 2003 [13]	—	126	34	25	51
Schelling *et al.* 2003 [34]	Cardiac surgery	148	—	—	18.2
Relatives					
Jones *et al.* (*in press* [16])	—	104	24	—	49

ARDS: acute respiratory distress syndrome.

Post-traumatic stress disorder – diagnosis

There are six obligatory diagnostic criteria (Box 5.1) [14]. The first important criterion requires exposure to either a traumatic event involving death, serious injury or a threat to themselves or others. The patient's response must involve intense fear, helplessness or horror. For relatives the experience of seeing the patient close to death and their own feelings of helplessness fulfils this criterion. For the patients themselves, it may not be a true perception of their illness but rather nightmares or hallucinations. For example, one patient remembered that she was trying to stop people abusing her daughter and she could not because she was given an injection to sedate her. Such experiences are described by patients as being real and hence difficult to dismiss afterwards.

PTSD is characterised by a range of symptoms such as re-experiencing the event (flashbacks), avoidance of situations that remind patients of the event, a numbed reaction and symptoms of increased arousal. PTSD can only be diagnosed when the symptoms have been present for more than 1 month. There are many tools for diagnosing and screening for PTSD [15]. However, only a small number have been used with ICU patients [16]. A short, easy to use tool indicating levels of symptoms requiring intervention (e.g. counselling or clinical psychology) would be useful. An early screening tool for use in clinic or over the telephone would be ideal. The PTSS-14 may be a suitable tool as it performed well in a pilot study [17]. The PTSS-14 is a short questionnaire covering 14 of the 17 symptoms of PTSD (Box 5.2). It takes 3–5 min to complete, making it suitable for

Box 5.1 *Diagnostic and Statistical Manual of Mental Disorders*-IV **Criteria for PTSD**

The following six diagnostic criteria must be met for a diagnosis of PTSD

1. The person has been exposed to a traumatic event in which both of the following were present:

   - The person experienced, witnessed, or was confronted with an event or events involving actual or threatened death or serious injury, or a threat to the physical integrity of self or others.
   - The persons' response involved intense fear, helplessness, or horror.

2. The traumatic event continues to be re-experienced in one or more of the following ways:

   - Recurrent and intrusive distressing recollections of the event, including images, thoughts, or perceptions.
   - Recurrent distressing dreams of the event.
   - Acting or feeling as if the traumatic event were recurring, including a sense of reliving the experience, illusions, hallucinations, and dissociative flashbacks which can occur on awakening, when intoxicated, or at other times.
   - Intense psychological distress at exposure to internal or external cues that symbolise or resemble an aspect of the traumatic event.
   - Physiologic reactivity on exposure to internal or external cues that symbolise or resemble an aspect of the traumatic event.

3. Persistent avoidance of stimuli associated with the trauma and numbing of general responsiveness which was not present before the trauma, including three or more of the following:

   - Efforts to avoid activities, places, or people that arouse recollections of the trauma.
   - Inability to recall an important aspect of the trauma.
   - Markedly diminished interest or participation in significant activities.

Continued on Page 43

- Feeling of detachment or estrangement from others.
- Restricted range of affect, for example, unable to have loving or angry feelings.
- Sense of a foreshortened future, for example, does not expect to have a career, marriage, children, or a normal life span.

4. Persistent symptoms of increased arousal, not present before the trauma, as indicated by two or more of the following:
   - Difficulty falling or staying asleep.
   - Irritability or outbursts of anger.
   - Difficulty concentrating.
   - Hypervigilance.
   - Exaggerated startle response.
5. Duration of the disturbance symptoms in 2, 3 and 4 for more than one month.
6. There is clinically significant distress or impairment in social, occupational, or other important areas of functioning.

outpatient clinic or telephone use. In the pilot study the PTSS-14 scores at 2 months predicted PTSD at 3 months using a full interview diagnostic tool.

Cognitive model

The way an individual processes information at the time of the traumatic event may be important in developing PTSD. Individuals who report feeling confused and overwhelmed as they experienced the traumatic situation are more likely to suffer from persistent PTSD [18,19]. These patients may lack perceptual processing of the traumatic situation (i.e. are unable to process the meaning in an organised way). Instead they will concentrate on processing sensory impressions of the situation; this is termed data-driven processing [20]. ICU patients may be more at risk of PTSD because, during the traumatic event, be it ICU treatment or critical illness itself, their ability to process information is compromised by factors such as critical illness, delirium, sleep deprivation and sedative drugs. There may be an association between the use of sedatives in ICU and PTSD symptoms at 6–41 months after ICU in patients recovering from adult respiratory distress syndrome (ARDS) [21] due to a reduced perceptual state.

Box 5.2 The PTSS-14 Questionnaire

This form should not take longer than about 5 minutes to complete. The form has two sections, Part A and Part B.

PART A

This consists of four statements about your memory of the time you spent on the Intensive Care Unit. Read each statement. If a statement is FALSE, tick the NO box. If the statement is TRUE, tick the YES box. Please answer ALL four questions. Tick only ONE box for each statement. If you make a mistake, simply cross out the wrong answer and tick the correct box.

PART B

This consists of 14 statements about how you have been feeling in the past few days. You need to decide HOW OFTEN you have been feeling this way in the past few days. If you have NOT EVER felt or experienced what the statement says in the past few days, circle 1 (never). If you have been feeling or experiencing it ALL THE TIME, circle 7 (always). Otherwise, circle one of the numbers in between that best describes how much you have been feeling or experiencing what the statement says in the past few days. Please circle only one number for each statement. If you make a mistake, simply cross it out and circle the correct number. PLEASE be sure to choose a number for ALL 14 statements.

A. When I think back to the time of my severe illness and the time I spent in the ICU, I remember:

Nightmares	No	Yes
Severe anxiety or panic	No	Yes
Severe pain	No	Yes
Troubles to breath, feelings of suffocation	No	Yes

B. Presently (this means in the past few days) I suffer from:

1. *sleep problems*

never   always

1	2	3	4	5	6	7

Continued on Page 45

2. *nightmares*

never   always

1   2   3   4   5   6   7

3. *depression, I feel dejected/downtrodden*

never   always

1   2   3   4   5   6   7

4. *jumpiness, I am easily frightened by sudden sounds or sudden movements*

never   always

1   2   3   4   5   6   7

5. *the need to withdraw from others*

never   always

1   2   3   4   5   6   7

6. *irritability, that is, I am easily agitated/annoyed and angry*

never   always

1   2   3   4   5   6   7

7. *frequent mood swings*

never   always

1   2   3   4   5   6   7

8. *a bad conscience, blame myself, have guilt feelings*

never   always

1   2   3   4   5   6   7

9. *fear of places and situations, which remind me of the Intensive Care Unit*

never   always

1   2   3   4   5   6   7

10. *muscular tension*

never   always

1   2   3   4   5   6   7

Continued on Page 46

Box 5.2

11. *upsetting, unwanted thoughts or images of my time on the Intensive Care Unit*

never   always

1   2   3   4   5   6   7

12. *feeling numb (e.g. cannot cry, unable to have loving feelings)*

never   always

1   2   3   4   5   6   7

13. *avoid places, people or situations that remind me of the Intensive Care Unit*

never   always

1   2   3   4   5   6   7

14. *feeling as if my plans or dreams for the future will not come true*

never   always

1   2   3   4   5   6   7

Neurocircuitry model

The amygdala, an almond-shaped structure in the brain situated just above the brainstem connecting the thalamus and cortex, seems to play a central role in PTSD [22]. The amygdala undertakes threat evaluation of incoming sensory information. The anterior cingulated cortex is an area in the prefrontal cortex that is connected to the amygdala and has a role in conditioned fear. An example of conditional fear is if your neighbour's dog bites you, then you are likely to be wary not just when you see the dog but every time you pass the neighbour's property. Extinction of this conditioned fear is when you are able to pass the house without developing the fear response, but still being able to remember the dog bite. The anterior cingulated cortex is activated less in patients suffering from PTSD compared to controls during symptom provocation [23]. It is not clear whether this reduced activation fails to inhibit an overactive amygdala when reminders of the traumatic event occur or whether the activation reduction is more generalised in patients with PTSD [24].

In addition, the hippocampus may be involved in PTSD; it plays a role in contextual fear. An example of contextual fear is where a rat escapes from a fox and becomes conditioned not only to the stimulus of the fox's presence but also where the event took place. For some intensive care patients, the ICU is a source of contextual fear. The hippocampus is also involved in the storage of incoming stimuli to longer-term memory. Several studies have found reduced hippocampal volume in PTSD patients. However, it is not clear whether this reduction was present before the PTSD or developed as a result of the symptoms. A study comparing two sets of identical twins suggests that smaller hippocampal volume may make individuals vulnerable to developing PTSD [25]. The impact of critical illness and sepsis on the brain is only just starting to be investigated. A recent study involving post-mortem examination of patients dying of septic shock showed cell death and ischaemia within the amygdala [26]. The intensity of apoptosis was correlated with endothelial expression of inducible nitric oxide synthase. Whether some degree of cell death and ischaemia can be seen in patients who survive a severe septic illness in ICU has not yet been examined.

Therapy

There will be a core of patients who will be overwhelmed by feelings of panic, intrusive memories of ICU or be unable to sleep due to recurrent nightmares. These patients find it very difficult to cope with the transition from ICU to the general ward and then to home. It is this group of patients who may benefit from early psychological intervention [27]. Interventions such as anxiety management (e.g. breathing control, muscle relaxation training and self-talk exercises) can be useful in controlling panic attacks. Controlled imaginal exposure to traumatic memories is thought to promote habituation [28]. For recurrent nightmares a different, positive ending to the dream can be practiced by the patient while awake, and this can, in some cases, change the nightmare. This technique called imagery rehearsal therapy has been shown to reduce chronic nightmares and improve sleep quality [29]. Anecdotally our own experience of early psychological interventions with ICU patients on the general wards does seem to have helped to reduce the need for later referral to clinical psychology.

Conclusion

Anxiety and panic attacks are common in recently discharged ICU patients. For many patients, these symptoms will be self-limited and resolve over a few days or weeks. However, some patients will require formal referral to psychiatric services. It is vital that these patients be identified early as this improves the prognosis. Relatives also suffer from PTSD after ICU. This is not surprising considering how traumatic their experiences are. In some cases, there may be a need for family therapy to allow the whole family to come to terms with their experience.

References

1. Shi SF, Munjas BA, Wan TT, Cowling WR, Grap MJ, Wang BB. The effects of preparatory sensory information on ICU patients. *J Med Syst* 2003;**27**:191–204.
2. Goldman LS, Kimball CP. Depression in intensive care units. *Int J Psychiatry Med* 1987;**17**:201–12.
3. Bardellini S, Servadio G, Chiarello M, Chiarello E. Sleep disorders in patients in recovery: preliminary results in 20 patients. *Minerva Anestesiol* 1992;**58**:527–33.
4. Chlan LL. Description of anxiety levels by individual differences and clinical factors in patients receiving mechanical ventilatory support. *Heart Lung* 2003;**32**:275–82.
5. House A, Mayou R, Mallinson C. *Psychiatric Aspects of Physical Disease*. London: Royal College of Physicians and Royal College of Psychiatrists, 1995, pp. 1–2.
6. McKinley S, Nagy S, Stein-Parbury J, Bramwell M, Hudson J. Vulnerability and security in seriously ill patients in intensive care. *Intens Crit Care Nurs* 2002;**18**:27–36.
7. Pochard F, Azoulay E, Chevret S, *et al.* Symptoms of anxiety and depression in family members of intensive care unit patients: ethical hypothesis regarding decision-making capacity. *Crit Care Med* 2001;**29**:2025–6.
8. Jones C, Griffiths RD. Social support and anxiety levels in relatives of critically ill patients. *Br J Intens Care* 1995;**5**:44–7.
9. Jones C, Skirrow P, Griffiths RD, *et al.* Post traumatic stress disorder-related symptoms in relatives of patients following intensive care. *Intens Care Med* 2004;**30**:456–60.
10. Tian ZM, Reis Miranda D. Quality of life after intensive care with the sickness impact profile. *Intens Care Med* 1995;**21**:422–8.
11. Jones C, Griffiths RD, Macmillan RR, Palmer TEA. Psychological problems occurring after intensive care. *Br J Intens Care* 1994;**4**:46–53.
12. Jones C, Griffiths RD, Humphris GH, Skirrow PM. Memory, delusions, and the development of acute posttraumatic stress disorder-related symptoms after intensive care. *Crit Care Med* 2001;**29**:573–80.
13. Jones C, Skirrow P, Griffiths RD, *et al.* Rehabilitation after critical illness: a randomised, controlled trial. *Crit Care Med* 2003;**31**:2456–61.
14. American Psychiatric Association. *Diagnostic and Statistical Manual of Mental Disorders*, 4th Edn., Text Revised. Washington, DC: American Psychiatric Association, 2000.
15. Foa EB, Keane TM, Friedman MJ. *Practical Guidelines from the International Society for Traumatic Stress Studies – Effective Treatments for PTSD*. New York: The Guilford Press, 2000.
16. Jones C, Twigg E, Lurie A, *et al.* The challenge of diagnosis of stress reactions following intensive care and early intervention: a review. *Clin Intens Care* (in press).

17. Twigg E, Jones C, McDougall M, Griffiths RD, Humphris GH. Early screening tool for post traumatic stress disorder following critical illness. *Br J Anaesth* 2003,**90**:540P.
18. Ehlers A, Clark DM. A cognitive model of posttraumatic stress disorder. *Behav Res Ther* 2000;**38**:319–45.
19. Dunmore E, Clark DM, Ehlers A. A prospective investigation of the role of cognitive factors in persistent posttraumatic stress disorder (PTSD) after physical or sexual assault. *Behav Res Ther* 2001;**39**:1063–84.
20. Murray J, Ehlers A, Mayou RA. Dissociation and post-traumatic stress disorder: two prospective studies of road traffic accident survivors. *Br J Psychiatry* 2002;**180**:363–8.
21. Nelson BJ, Weinert CR, Bury CL, Marinelli WA, Gross CR. Intensive care unit drug use and subsequent quality of life in acute lung injury patients. *Crit Care Med* 2000;**28**:3626–30.
22. LeDoux J. Brain mechanisms of emotion and emotional learning. *Curr Opin Neurobiol* 1992;**2**:191–7.
23. Bremner JD, Narayan M, Staib LH, *et al.* Neural correlates of memories of childhood sexual abuse in women with and without posttraumatic stress disorder. *Arch Gen Psychiatry* 1997;**54**:246–56.
24. Tanev K. Neuroimaging and neurocircuitry in post-traumatic stress disorder: what is currently known. *Curr Psychiatric Reports* 2003;**5**:369–83.
25. Gilbertson MW, Shenton ME, Ciszewski A, *et al.* Smaller hippocampal volume predicts pathological vulnerability to psychological trauma. *Nat Neurosci* 2002;**5**:1242–7.
26. Sharshar T, Gray F, Lorin de la Grandmaison G, *et al.* Apoptosis of neurons in cardiovascular autonomic centres triggered by inducible nitric oxide synthase after death from septic shock. *Lancet* 2003;**362**:1799–1805.
27. Rothbaum BO, Mellman TA. Dreams and exposure therapy in PTSD. *J Trauma Stress* 2001;**14**:481–90.
28. Forbes D, Phelps AJ, McHugh AF, Debenham P, Hopwood M, Creamer M. Imagery rehearsal in the treatment of posttraumatic nightmares in Australian veterans with chronic combat-related PTSD: 12-month follow-up data. *J Trauma Stress* 2003;**16**:509–13.
29. Koshy G, Wilkinson A, Harmsworth A, Waldmann CS. Intensive care unit follow-up program at a district general hospital. *Intens Care Med* 1997;**23**:S160.
30. Schelling G, Stoll C, Meier M, *et al.* Health-related quality of life and post-traumatic stress disorder in survivors of adult respiratory distress syndrome. *Crit Care Med* 1998;**26**:651–9.
31. Nelson BJ, Weinert CR, Bury CL, Marinelli WA, Gross CR. Intensive care unit drug use and subsequent quality of life in acute lung injury patients. *Crit Care Med* 2000;**28**:3626–30.
32. Schnyder U, Moergeli H, Klaghofer R, Buddeberg C. Incidence and prediction of posttraumatic stress disorder symptoms in severely injured accident victims. *Am J Psychiatry* 2001;**158**:594–9.
33. Scragg P, Jones A, Fauvel N. Psychological problems following ICU treatment. *Anaesthesia* 2001;**56**:9–14.
34. Schelling G, Richter M, Roozendal B, *et al.* Exposure to high stress in the intensive care unit may have negative effects on health-related quality-of-life outcomes after cardiac surgery. *Crit Care Med* 2003;**31**:1971–80.

6: The impact of admission to paediatric intensive care unit (PICU) on the child and family

GILLIAN COLVILLE

Introduction

The admission of a child to a paediatric intensive care unit (PICU) is, even when planned, a source of considerable anxiety for parents. An emergency admission represents a crisis for a family. There are suddenly many potential losses to be faced such as disfigurement, brain damage and, most feared of all, death. On PICU parents may, for the first time, be told a child's diagnosis. This can sometimes have catastrophic implications for the rest of the family, for example, if a baby is found to have a degenerative genetic condition or to be human immunodeficiency virus (HIV) positive. Initial relief that a child has survived may be replaced by the awful realisation that he or she will never be the same again. For some families, there is significant strain associated with the uncertainty of prognosis or increased dependency placed on the parent–child relationship, by the demands of chronic illness.

On admission the child may be very frightened by the deterioration in his or her condition and bewildered by the rising anxiety evident in their parents. On the unit they will often be subjected to numerous invasive procedures such as cannulation and suctioning. As they recover they may experience disturbing side-effects as their sedation is weaned and they become more aware of the distress of other patients and their families.

In 1993, the British Paediatric Association recommended that the special psychosocial needs of children on PICUs and their families be addressed [1]. However, 5 years later only 54% of paediatric units in the UK had a social worker on their staff. Only 31% of PICUs were supported by a psychologist and 19% had no dedicated psychosocial staff [2]. In practice, therefore, the job of addressing families' psychological needs mainly falls to the medical and nursing staff.

Literature on parents' experiences of intensive care

There is evidence that, during an admission to intensive care, significant numbers of relatives suffer symptoms of anxiety and depression [3]; however, there is little information on how long these symptoms persist after discharge. Higher levels of anxiety are reported in relatives with lower rates of contact with medical staff, and as many as half have problems understanding the patient's diagnosis [4]. Also, the effectiveness of interventions designed to tackle communication problems is unknown.

In a comprehensive review of studies of parents' experiences and needs while on PICU, Noyes [5] found that the data were predominantly quantitative, written from a nursing perspective and North American in origin. Youngblut and Jay [6] identified the following areas as giving rise to the highest levels of concern: the child's survival, the possibility of brain damage, seeing the child in pain and the diagnosis. The environmental assault of ICUs on the senses (referred to as 'sensoristrain' by Black, Deeny and McKenna [7]) has been assumed to exacerbate parents' distress. However, the principal finding of Carter and Miles' work [8] was that the main strain for parents was the disruption of their parental role, with mothers exhibiting higher levels of stress than fathers [9] (Figure 6.1). Furthermore, it has been demonstrated that stress-related symptoms in mothers persist for months after discharge and are consistently higher than those of mothers of children admitted to a general ward [10]. Lastly although there is

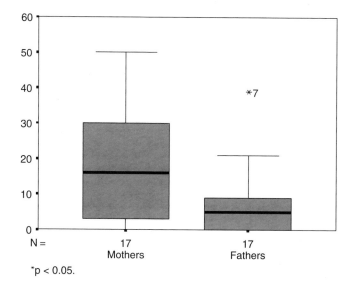

Figure 6.1 Mothers' and fathers' scores on the Impact of Events Scale (IES). Scale scores reflect number of post-traumatic stress symptoms, with scores over 20 regarded as clinically significant and scores over 35 suggestive of full post-traumatic stress disorder (PTSD).

Box 6.1 The reported positive aspects of parents' experience on PICU

- 'Because of the accident, he is very, very, special to me'
- 'We saw the best of people during that time'
- 'I re-valued my life totally. This house could burn down tomorrow as long as my family stood out there I wouldn't worry'

---

evidence that parents' memories of events during admission remain vivid for a long time after discharge [11,12], it is important to be aware that parents report positive as well as negative experiences and, in the longer term, the majority cope remarkably well [13] (Box 6.1).

Literature on the child's experience of intensive care

The literature on adult survivors of critical care contains descriptions of distressing memories relating to painful and frightening experiences, including fear of death and the inability to communicate while intubated [14]. Much less is known about the experience of children in this situation. Distress in a conscious child during admission may present as marked lack of engagement or as active resistance. The latter directly impacts on the child's medical condition; an anxious child may resist mechanical ventilation, and associated increases in heart and metabolic rate place further demands on an already critically ill patient. Ambuel et al. [15] point out the limitations of many commonly used behavioural distress scales (which are primarily intended to measure acute pain in relation to discrete procedures) when applied to this population. They have developed a useful observational scoring system for measuring distress in the PICU setting (the COMFORT Scale), which takes account of the child's limited opportunity to communicate or move, and which can be used for continuous observation.

Post-traumatic stress symptoms have been described in three children following intubation [16], as well as 'out of body' or 'near death' experiences [17]. The quality of sleep on intensive care is another issue that has been examined on PICU. Normal sleep stages are not seen and rapid eye movement sleep is absent [18]. Playfor [19] found that only 60% of children remembered their admission, and that their memories were predominantly neutral or positive (Box 6.2 and Figure 6.2). However, two more recent studies [20,21], which employed standardised psychological measures and followed up children over a longer period, have reported significant levels of post-traumatic stress in survivors of PICU.

Box 6.2 The reported views of children after PICU admission

- 'I am not as scared as I was – now when I get a cut it is just nothing'
- 'I think I am a bit more grown up'
- 'I feel like I am the odd one out of everybody'
- 'I really miss the way I was before'

What I remember about PICU

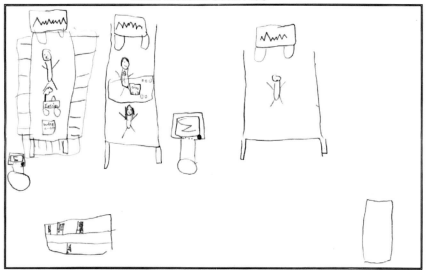

Figure 6.2 A child's perspective of PICU.

A recent study [22] exploring the hospital experiences of a group of ventilator-dependent children concluded that prolonged PICU admission has a 'profound and negative impact' on the quality of life of this particular subgroup of patients who may require more psychosocial input [23]. The fact that such children are often more aware of what is going on around them than other patients on PICU means that they are more likely to be affected emotionally by separations from family, by having multiple carers, and being at much greater risk of witnessing untoward events [24]. An increasing number of these patients are spending long periods in intensive care because of practical problems arranging discharge [25].

Research on parents at St George's

In order to establish the degree of psychological distress in parents follow-ing their child's admission to PICU, and identify factors associated with poor psychological adjustment, 52 parents were interviewed about their memories of PICU and current psychological functioning, 8 months after discharge. Measures included the Parental Stressor Scale (PSS: PICU) [8], the General Health Questionnaire-28 (GHQ-28) [26] and the Impact of Events Scale (IES) [27]. Significant rates of psychological distress were found, with 60% of the sample scoring above accepted cut-offs on either GHQ-28 or IES. Distress was not associated with child demographic or medical variables but was associated with subjective rates of stress during admission as measured by the PSS: PICU (Figure 6.3). Parents who talked about their feelings at the time of the admission had lower IES scores at 8 months than those who did not; the majority of parents would have appre-ciated the offer of a follow-up appointment [28]. Parents who wanted an appointment reported higher scores on PSS: PICU and IES than those who did not (Box 6.3). Although satisfaction with care on PICU was generally high, parents frequently described harrowing experiences before admission (echoing comments from a previous study evaluating parents' experience of patient retrieval [29]) and afterwards on the general wards. Where data

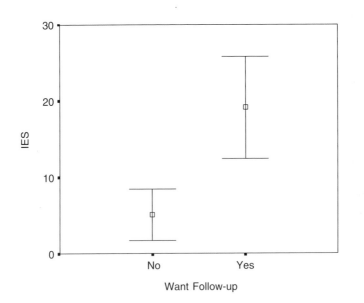

Figure 6.3 Distress levels in parents (n = 52) as measured by their responses to the Impact of Events Scale (IES) scores, divided into parents who did or did not want follow-up support. The threshold value for clinical concern is 20.

Box 6.3 Dimensions measured by the Parental Stressor Scale (PSS): PICU

- Child's appearance
- Procedures
- Sights and sounds
- Staff behaviour
- Parental roles
- Child's emotional and behavioural responses
- Staff communication

---

were available for both parents, mothers reported significantly higher rates of distress at follow up than fathers [30].

Given the finding that a significant proportion of families would appreciate further contact after their child's admission, it was decided in a subsequent prospective study, to offer a follow-up clinic appointment with PICU staff randomly to half a cohort of families of surviving children over the course of 1 year. Preliminary results suggest that although these appointments have been well received when parents have taken them up, only a minority of families have chosen to attend. Ongoing analyses will examine differences between those who attended and those who did not and explore the reasons for non-attendance.

Research on children at St George's

The author has examined two sources of information regarding children's experience of PICU: parents' reports of the degree to which they felt their child had been affected by the experience of being admitted to PICU [31] and direct interviews with a cohort of children aged over 7 years [32].

In the first study, the mothers of 48 children were asked, as part of a semi-structured interview 8 months after their child's discharge, about the impact of PICU admission on their children. Those parents whose children were aged over 2 years ($n = 22$) also completed a standardised behaviour questionniare on their child's current psychological functioning [33].

Only 8 out of 48 mothers felt their child had been changed by the experience, with 10 out of 12 parents of children under 1 year, feeling the question was not applicable because of their child's age. However, 29 parents reported that their relationship with the child had changed. Parents described feeling closer to the child but also frequently fearful about the child's well-being. Most parents acknowledged that their relationship has been altered by experience of PICU and were aware of continuing to be overprotective many months after the child was out of danger – a phenomenon well recognised by paediatricians in parents of children who have survived serious illness [34]. However, the children's distribution of scores on the behaviour questionnaire was normal, indicating that they were not exhibiting significant behaviour problems.

In the second interview study, 15 children were asked what they remembered of their admission to PICU and how much they still felt affected 9 months later, by which time they had usually recovered physically and were able to reflect on the experience. Standardised psychological questionnaires were administered: the child version of the IES [35], the Birleson Child Depression Scale [36] and the Fear Survey Schedule for Children (FSSC) [37]. Interviews were held 9 months after discharge and in addition parents completed the Achenbach Child Behaviour Checklist (CBCL).

Although, as in the previous study, parents did not rate the children as having significant behaviour problems, six children scored in the clinically significant range on one or more measures, during direct interviewing. These conflicting results suggest there is a need for further research on the child's experience, and demonstrate that parents may not always be aware of the extent to which their child has been affected by their admission. Lastly, the way children responded to the FSSC was surprising in that they reported significantly fewer fears than age- and sex-matched peers. It is possible that this finding reflected the fact that only the most constitutionally resilient of children were prepared to be interviewed. It may however be a genuine reaction to surviving trauma, as some children clearly articulated during the interview.

Clinical implications

The scope for preparation is limited, given the acute nature of many admissions, but where admission to PICU is planned, it may be possible to introduce both child and family to the unit beforehand. Knowledge gained about the anxieties of the family at this stage may usefully inform future involvement with the family. For example, past negative associations with the intensive care environment need to be taken into account in understanding the special significance of an admission, however routine from the staff's point of view.

The main reasons for referral to the paediatric psychologist during an admission centre around management of the child's distress, communication and occupation. The procedures to which children are subjected whilst in intensive care are inevitably distressing and painful. Thus, good pain control is essential, particularly where a child is conscious; an effort should be made to schedule invasive procedures in such a way as to minimise distress [38]. It has been demonstrated that where PICU patients are 'conscious but markedly non-engaged', the introduction of age-appropriate activities increased positive affect and decreased inappropriate behaviours such as self-stimulation and interfering with medical equipment. Another simple intervention where a young child was given an environmental cue in the form of a red light (which was switched on whenever an invasive procedure was imminent) brought about a marked reduction in overall anxiety [39].

A child with some awareness of their surroundings on PICU may well become fearful while anticipating a procedure. This might be because they know from experience that it will be painful, or because they are so bewildered that they do not trust anyone. The well-established principles of desensitisation and adapting interventions to take account of the child's interests apply. A child may be referred for being uncooperative (e.g. for spitting into the nurse's eye whenever she attempts suction of secretions from the tracheotomy). In such a case, it can be very helpful to understand this behaviour in the context of the child's need for control over a situation where he or she feels overwhelmingly powerless, and where possible, adjust some of the parameters of PICU management accordingly.

In contrast to most patients on PICU, children who are ventilator-dependent may be fully conscious of what is going on around them and may be on the unit for some time. If available, the skills of a play therapist are often invaluable with these children. Advice should be provided on developmental appropriateness of play materials and the need for the children to gain some control over their surroundings. The usual pastimes of listening to stories or musical tapes and watching videos will soothe and lift a child's mood in the short term, but during longer admissions more varied materials should be offered, in the interests of the child's overall development and emotional well-being. A paraplegic child can derive all the usual pleasure afforded by doll play, if someone is on hand to follow his or her instructions. There is also a particular delight to be watching another messing around with paints, in this sterile, orderly environment.

For a significant number of parents, any discussion of their own emotional state whilst their child's medical condition is critical is simply too painful and regarded by them as an unwanted distraction. At this acute stage it is important to respect the parents' need to hold themselves together by whatever individual coping strategies they find helpful in the short term. Contact may consist of little more than gentle reminders to take breaks, sleep and eat, and an opportunity to discuss the logistics of visiting arrangements. There is also a place for providing normalising information describing how other parents have felt in similar circumstances. Advice may be sought as to whether siblings should be allowed to visit and about what they should be told. Parents may also seek guidance on how to handle a sibling's attention-seeking behaviour or separation distress.

It is often after transfer from intensive care to the general ward that the child's distress is most apparent. As the sedation wears off they become

---

Box 6.4 Parents' comments about their child's appearance

- 'She looked totally drugged, dazed, gone, she was just out, puffy'
- 'She just looked horrific, bright red face, tubes coming out of every possible place'
- 'She was so bloated and she looked terrible, I just could not make myself to go near her'

---

more aware of pain and begin to try to make sense of what has happened. At this point they may experience nightmares or hallucinations and be uncharacteristically wary and fearful. The side-effects of weaning off morphine and midazolam may temporarily render the child unrecognisable to close family [40] (Box 6.4). This can be very upsetting for parents who may be anxiously seeking evidence that the child is returning to normal, particularly if there has been any question of brain damage. Even if the child is not unduly distressed, there may be some value in a psychologist making contact with a family, where the circumstances that gave rise to the admission are known to have been traumatic. Information can be given, both about normal reactions after an accident and how to seek further support.

Subsequent involvement, after discharge, may take the form of intervention focusing on post-traumatic stress symptoms, help with newly acquired fears, particularly around further medical treatment or providing general support for the child and family. Older children sometimes appreciate being provided with a list of operations, giving names of procedures and dates performed, as they piece together details that are otherwise confused and sketchy.

Parents sometimes present clinically to the psychology service months later claiming that the relationship with their child has altered irrevocably since admission. They describe being aware of the fate of other children who died on the unit and report something akin to survivor guilt, albeit by proxy, which is experienced as especially troubling. In common with other trauma survivors, they no longer feel the world is a safe place and lose confidence in their ability to tell whether a child is ill or not, leading to increased rates of consulting behaviour both in primary and secondary health care settings.

Conclusion

It is important to strike a balance between acknowledging the strain on families on PICU and 'over-pathologising' their reactions. Whilst it is clear that the admission of a child to PICU is often experienced as traumatic, for the most part it does not lead to severe psychological distress. More research is needed on the natural history of stress reactions in parents and children in this setting and into ways of identifying those at highest risk of developing long-term problems, in order that appropriate timely support can be offered to those most in need.

Acknowledgements

The author's research was funded by St George's Charitable Foundation and the Paediatric Intensive Care Society.

References

1. British Paediatric Association. *The Care of Critically Ill Children*. London: British Paediatric Association, 1993.
2. Colville G. Psychosocial support on the paediatric intensive care unit: a UK survey. *Care of the Crit Ill* 1998;**14**:25–8.
3. Pochard F, Azoulay E, Chevret S, *et al*. Symptoms of anxiety and depression in family members of intensive care unit patients: ethical hypothesis regarding decision-making capacity. *Crit Care Med* 2001;**29**:1893–7.
4. Azoulay E, Chevret S, Lelen G, *et al*. Half the families of intensive care unit patients experience inadequate communication with physicians. *Crit Care Med* 2000;**28**:3044–9.
5. Noyes J. A critique of studies exploring the experiences and needs of parents of children admitted to paediatric intensive care units. *J Adv Nurs* 1998;**28**:134–42.
6. Youngblut JM, Jay SS. Emergent admission to the pediatric intensive care unit: parental concerns. *AACN Clin Issues Crit Care Nurs* 1991;**2**:329–37.
7. Black P, Deeny P, McKenna H. Sensoristrain: an exploration of nursing interventions in the context of the Neuman systems theory. *Intens Crit Care Nurs* 1997;**13**:249–58.
8. Carter MC, Miles MS. The Parental Stressor Scale: pediatric intensive care unit. *Matern Child Nurs J* 1989;**18**:187–98.
9. Riddle II, Hennessey J, Eberly TW, Carter MC, Miles MS. Stressors in the pediatric intensive care unit as perceived by mothers and fathers. *Matern Child Nurs J* 1989;**18**:221–34.
10. Board R, Ryan-Wenger N. Stressors and stress symptoms of mothers with children in the PICU. *J Pediatr Nurs* 2003;**18**:195–202.
11. Meyer EC, Garcia Coll CT, Seifer R, Ramos A, Kilis E, Oh W. Psychological distress in mothers of preterm infants. *J Dev Behav Pediatr* 1995;**16**:412–7.
12. Wereszczak J, Miles MS, Holditch-Davis D. Maternal recall of the neonatal intensive care unit. *Neonatal Netw* 1997;**16**:33–40.
13. Affleck G, Tennen H, Rowe J. *Infants in Crisis: How Parents Cope with Newborn Intensive Care and its Aftermath*. New York: Springer-Verlag, 1991.
14. Menzel LK. Factors related to the emotional responses of intubated patients to being unable to speak. *Heart Lung* 1998;**27**:245–52.

15. Ambuel B, Hamlett KW, Marx XM, Burmer JL. Assessing distress in paediatric intensive care environments: the COMFORT scale. *J Pediatr Psychol* 1992;**17**:95–109.
16. Gavin LA, Roesler TA. Posttraumatic distress in children and families after intubation. *Pediatr Emerg Care* 1997;**13**:222–4.
17. Morse ML. Near-death experiences of children. *J Pediatr Oncol Nurs* 1994;**11**:139–44.
18. Donnelly JA, Cullen P, Morrison CM. Sleep in paediatric intensive care. *Care of the Crit Ill* 1997;**13**:163.
19. Playfor S, Thomas D, Choonara I. Recollection of children following intensive care. *Arch Dis Child* 2000;**83**: 445–8.
20. Rennick JE, Johnston CC, Dougherty G, Platt R, Ritchie JA. Children's psychological responses after critical illness and exposure to invasive technology. *J Dev Behav Pediatr* 2002;**23**:133–44.
21. Judge D, Nadel S, Vergnaud S, Garralda ME. Psychiatric adjustment following meningococcal disease treated on a PICU. *Intens Care Med* 2002;**28**:648–50.
22. Noyes J. Enabling young 'ventilator-dependent' people to express their views and experiences of their care in hospital. *J Adv Nurs* 2000;**31**:1206–15.
23. Colville GA, Mok Q. Psychological management of two cases of self-injury on the paediatric intensive care unit. *Arch Dis Child* 2003;**88**:335–6.
24. Gemke RJ, Bonsel GJ, van Vught AJ. Long-term survival and state of health after paediatric intensive care. *Arch Dis Child* 1995;**73**:196–201.
25. Fraser J, Mok Q, Tasker R. Survey of occupancy of paediatric intensive care units by children who are dependent on ventilators. *Br Med J* 1997;**315**:347–8.
26. Goldberg DP, Hillier VF. A scaled version of the General Health Questionnaire. *Psychol Med* 1979;**9**:139–45.
27. Horowitz MJ, Wilner N, Alvarez W. Impact of Event Scale: a measure of subjective stress. *Psychosom Med* 1979;**41**:209–18.
28. Colville GA, Cream PR, Gracey D. Parents' views on follow-up after paediatric intensive care. *Br J Anaesth* 2003;**90**:548P.
29. Colville G, Orr F, Gracey D. 'The worst journey of our lives': parents' experiences of a specialist retrieval service. *Intens Crit Care Nurs* 2003;**19**:103–8.
30. Colville GA, Cream PR, Gracey D. Psychological reactions of parents after paediatric intensive care: differences between mothers and fathers. *Br J Anaesth* 2003;**90**:548P–9P.
31. Colville G. Parents' views on the psychological impact of admission to paediatric intensive care. *Eur Psychother* 2004;**4**:81.
32. Colville G. Children's views on the psychological impact of admission to paediatric intensive care. *Eur Psychother* 2004;**4**:80.
33. Achenbach TM. *Integrative Guide for the 1991 CBCL/4-18, YSR, and RF Profiles*. Burlington, Vermont: Department of Psychiatry, University of Vermont, 1991.
34. Green M, Solnit AJ. Reactions to the threatened loss of a child: a vulnerable child syndrome. *Pediatrics* 1964;**34**:58–66.
35. Yule W. Children's Impact of Events Scale (IES). In: Sclare I. ed. *Child Psychology Portfolio: Anxiety, Depression and Post-Traumatic Stress in Childhood.* Berkshire: National Foundation for Educational Research (NFER-Nelson), 1997.
36. Birleson P, Hudson I, Buchanan DG, Wolff S. Clinical evaluation of a self-rating scale for depressive disorder in childhood. *J Child Psychol Psychiatr* 1987;**28**:43–60.
37. Ollendick T. Reliability and validity of the Revised Fear Schedule for Children (FSSC-R). *Behav Res Ther* 1983;**21**:685–92.

38. Southall DP, Crown BC, Hartmann H, Harrison-Sewell C, Samuels MP. Invasive procedures in children receiving intensive care. *Br Med J* 1993; **306**:1512–3.
39. Cataldo MF, Bessman CA, Parker LH, Pearson JER, Rogers MC. Behavioural assessment for paediatric intensive care units. *J App Behav Anal* 1979; **12**:83–97.
40. Hughes J, Choonara I. Parental anxiety due to abnormal behaviour following withdrawal of sedation. *Intens Crit Care Nurs* 1998;**4**:8–10.

7: Cognitive impairment and consequences for recovery

STEPHEN BRETT

Introduction

The follow-up of survivors of critical illness by the staff who cared for them whilst they were unwell is a relatively new phenomenon, and, as part of critical care delivery, remains very much a minority activity. Primary teams, in hectic outpatient departments, review most patients with little opportunity to explore beyond the major active clinical problems. Recently, however, groups of intensive care clinicians have initiated follow-up clinics and have started to unearth a whole variety of problems that may form a part of the normal convalescence from critical illness. Cognitive dysfunction is one of these problems. Cognition is defined by the Oxford English Dictionary [1] as:

The mental action or process of acquiring knowledge through thought, experience, and the senses – a perception, sensation, or intuition resulting from this.

'Cognitive function' can be regarded as a generic term encompassing various aspects of intellectual activity including memory, attention and concentration, linguistic and numerical skills and executive function, which describes our ability to assimilate information, plan and respond. These aspects of intellectual functioning are clearly essential to high-quality independent existence.

In addition to cognitive dysfunction, the non-physical consequences of critical illness include symptoms of anxiety and depression, acute stress reactions and post-traumatic stress disorder (PTSD), social isolation and disruption of personal relationships [2,4,5,6]. Furthermore, critical illnesses such as head injury, stroke or cardiac arrest may produce direct brain injury, as can certain surgical procedures, in particular those involving cardiopulmonary bypass. In an individual, all of these non-physical and physical factors interact and can produce an important impact on quality of life [7].

Approximately 30% of patients attending the Hammersmith Hospital intensive care unit (ICU) follow-up clinic 3 months after ICU discharge complain of difficulties with concentration, short-term memory and with ability to undertake the simple mental tasks required for daily life. This is often echoed by accompanying family members. Thirty percent have similar figures to those reported by other studies discussed in detail later in this chapter. These difficulties represent an important burden impairing complete recovery.

Cognitive dysfunction after surgery and anaesthesia

A major challenge in understanding the origin of these symptoms is disentangling the impact of surgery and anaesthesia that many patients have experienced from that of critical illness. Such cognitive dysfunction is particularly apparent in the elderly and is reviewed by Dodds and Allison [8]. The underlying pathological mechanisms remain elusive, but the central impact of cholinergic drugs (particularly atropine) has been raised as a possible trigger.

The International Study of Postoperative Cognitive Dysfunction (ISPOCD) was a multinational study that enrolled 1218 patients (>60 years of age) prior to elective non-cardiac surgery [9]. Study subjects completed an extensive battery of neuropsychological tests, which was repeated at 7 days (or hospital discharge, if earlier) and at 3 months post-operatively. The investigators were particularly interested in hypotension and hypoxaemia. Thus, blood pressure was recorded every 15–30 minutes on the first post-operative night while peripheral pulse oximetry was measured continuously from the day of operation for the first 3 nights. Overall 25.8% (95% Confidence Intervals (CI) in 23.1–28.5%) of patients met criteria for cognitive dysfunction at the first post-operative assessment. At 3 months 9.9% (95% CI in 8.1–12%) still demonstrated cognitive impairment. A cohort of entry criteria-matched non-operated control subjects was also recruited (by advertisement), of whom 3.3% met the impairment criteria at first testing and 2.8% on re-testing. Neither hypoxaemia nor hypotension proved to be risk factors at any time. Age, duration of anaesthesia, educational level and post-operative complications were risk factors for early dysfunction, but only increasing age was a risk factor for dysfunction at 3 months. Thus for non-cardiac surgery, we would expect around 10% of elderly patients to manifest cognitive dysfunction.

Data from studies into the effects of carotid endarterectomy are rather complicated. Heyer *et al.* studied 102 patients undergoing carotid endarterectomy of whom 76 were studied again at 1 month and 33 at 5 months [10]. Eighty percent of patients demonstrated a decline in one or more psychometric tests immediately post-operatively but 60% demonstrated an *improvement* in one or more scores. During follow-up the overall picture was one of gradual improvement. The authors postulated that immediate declines were due to ischaemia or embolic phenomena, whereas improvements were due to better cerebral perfusion. The same group subsequently attempted to examine the impact of anaesthesia by repeating the study [11], but with the addition of a comparator group of patients who received the same anaesthetic but had spinal surgery (carotid endarterectomy $n = 80$, spinal surgery $n = 25$). A neuropsychological test battery was administered before surgery and at 1 and 30 days post-operatively. Overall there was a clear excess in morbidity in the carotid endarterectomy group immediately, and this was still apparent at 30 days. This was still significant in spite of a proportion of patients not attending for follow-up. Bizarrely, control patients of shorter stature were more likely to return for follow-up than taller ones.

Morbidity and mortality after cardiac surgery has been extensively investigated, and surgical and anaesthetic techniques designed specifically to minimise the impact on cognitive function have been developed. Recent epidemiological data are therefore of interest. Roach *et al.* conducted a prospective evaluation of 2108 patients undergoing surgery in one of 24 American institutions [12]. Adverse neurological outcomes were characterised as Type I (3.1% – focal injury, coma or stupor at discharge) or Type II (3% – deterioration in intellectual function, memory deficit or seizures). The in-hospital mortality was 21% for Type I outcomes, 10% for Type II outcomes and 2% for those with no adverse neurological outcome ($p < 0.001$). Lengths of stay were 25 days, 21 days, and 10 days ($p < 0.001$), and discharge to long-term facilities occurred in 69%, 39% and 10% of cases respectively ($p < 0.001$). Thus even 'modest' injury, that is, to intellectual function, is associated with a significant impact in terms of mortality and subsequent independent existence.

The deficits in cognitive function seem related to direct physical damage to brain tissue occurring during bypass. Kilminster *et al.* studied this relationship by measuring serum S-100, a protein released by damaged brain tissue, in 130 patients undergoing cardiac surgery [13]. These investigators found a mixed pattern of improvement and deficit in neuropsychological tests in their patients; anxiety and depression scores improved post-operatively, as did the results of a general health questionnaire. However, less S-100 release was associated with better neuropsychological performance, greater release being associated with age and longer bypass time.

The complexity of this subject was demonstrated by a 5-year longitudinal study. Two hundred and sixty-one patients were tested pre-operatively, before discharge, at 6 weeks, 6 months and at 5 years post-operatively [14]. Overall cognitive decline was evident in 36% at 6 weeks; this figure improved by 6 months, but was worse at 5 years. This was because those discharged without cognitive decline improved initially demonstrating a learning effect; however, patients who were discharged with impairment fared a lot worse (Figure 7.1).

Van Dijk *et al.* grouped 23 similar studies together to produce an overall estimate that 22.5% (95% CI in 18.7–26.4%) of patients exhibited cognitive decline at 2 months after cardiac surgery [15]. These authors

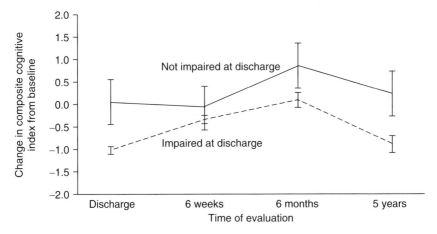

Figure 7.1 Composite cognitive index as a function of cognitive impairment at discharge. The composite cognitive index is the sum of four separate domain scores, and so provides an overview of cognitive performance, and thus may represent improvement in some areas as well as decline in others. Error bars represent standard error. From Newman et al. [14] with permission.

concluded by saying that an evaluation of the impact of 'off-pump' bypass grafting was needed and a number of such studies have now been published. Sixty patients were randomised by Zamvar *et al.* in a study specifically designed to detect an improvement using the off-pump technique and a standard test battery administered by a blinded investigator [16]. Overall, at 10 weeks post-operatively the incidence of impairment was high (40% in the bypass group); the off-pump group fared better with an incidence of 10% ($p < 0.017$). A Dutch study randomised 281 patients, of whom 249 were available for testing at 3 months [17]. The incidence of cognitive decline was 21% in the off-pump group and 29% in the on-pump group (relative risk 0.65, 95% CI in 0.36–1.16%, $p = 0.15$). At 1 year, the difference between the groups was less and there were no significant differences in quality of life, stroke rate or all-cause mortality. Other studies have similarly shown variable results [18,19].

Overall, therefore, critically ill post-operative patients come from a population already subjected to a substantial burden of cognitive decline. This is likely to be especially important in the very elderly and those requiring prolonged intensive care after cardiac surgery.

Psychological problems after critical illness

As mentioned earlier, a wide variety of non-physical problems have been described during recovery from critical illness, including affective disorders [2], symptoms consistent with PTSD [3] and more recently, cognitive dysfunction [20,21]. The best-characterised patient group is that of survivors of acute lung injury. Herridge *et al.* recently described the burden of continuing physical ill health at 1 year [22]. The performance of neuropsychological test batteries is mentally and physically demanding. Poor physical condition and affective state may exert an independent influence on performance of cognitive function testing; a number of studies on quality of life have revealed low scores for energy and vitality in critical care survivors [23,24,25,26]. Thus, in our own work we have selected a group of tests that can be administered in around 1 hour in an attempt to minimise subject fatigue (Figure 7.2).

Hopkins studied 55 survivors of the acute respiratory distress syndrome (ARDS) at hospital discharge and at 1 year [20]. A variety of outcomes were studied including quality of life, assessed with the Short Form-36 and the Sickness Impact Profile, and cognitive function assessed with an extensive range of tests administered by a trained psychologist. The particular aspects of cognitive function assessed were attention, memory, intelligence, processing speed, visuospatial skills and executive function. All patients

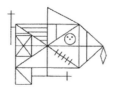

Asked to copy above picture, results below:

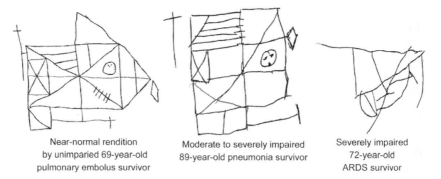

| Near-normal rendition by unimparied 69-year-old pulmonary embolus survivor | Moderate to severely impaired 89-year-old pneumonia survivor | Severely impaired 72-year-old ARDS survivor |

Figure 7.2 Rey–Osterrieth Complex Figure. A test of visuo-construction, in which the patient is asked to copy a complex geometric design, was administered to all patients 6 months after hospital discharge as a component of the neuropsychological battery of tests. This figure shows the original Rey–Osterrieth Complex Figure and the examples from three patients (all of whom had no detectable baseline cognitive deficits) as a visual depiction of the character of deficits found in the study cohort. Reproduced by special permission of the Publisher, Psychological Assessment Resources, Inc., 16204 North Florida Avenue, Lutz, FL 33549, from the Rey Complex Figure Test and Recognition Trial by John E. Meyers, Kelly R. Meyers. Copyright 1992 by Psychological Assessment Resources, Inc. Further reproduction is prohibited without permission of Psychological Assessment Resources, Inc. From Jackson et al. [21] with permission.

had clear evidence of widespread cognitive decline at hospital discharge. At 1 year, there was general improvement but 78% still exhibited evidence of impairment of one or more cognitive domains. The amount of time patients spent with low haemoglobin oxygen saturation during their acute illness was significantly correlated with impaired cognitive function. Moreover, the PaO_2 at study enrollment was significantly correlated with persisting dysfunction in several cognitive domains at 1 year but particularly memory. Cognitive dysfunction has been described in other diseases characterised by hypoxaemia, such as chronic obstructive pulmonary disease [27] and obstructive sleep apnoea [28].

Although Hopkins' study described a quality-of-life impact, it was unable to relate this to the degree of cognitive dysfunction. Rothenhäusler studied 46 patients at a median time of 6 years after survival from ARDS [29]. No patient had gross 'brain damage'. However, all of the patients exhibiting more subtle cognitive dysfunction were registered as disabled, compared with only a quarter of the unimpaired. Acute descriptors of illness severity were not related to cognitive outcome, suggesting that cognitive dysfunction is not simply a reflection of illness severity. Preliminary data from our own studies have also failed to demonstrate any link between acute illness severity and cognitive impairment, affective disorder or indeed subsequent quality of life [30].

Recently, Jackson et al. have described the impact of critical illness on cognitive function in a medical intensive care population [21]. Using strict criteria, one-third of patients were defined as neuropsychologically impaired at 6 months after ICU discharge. Although impaired patients had similar quality-of-life scores, depression scores were worse. The rate of cognitive deficits was greater than the 'norms' for a population with mild dementia. The authors compared the levels of dementia described with standard behavioural rating scales and concluded that patients exhibiting these levels of impairment would have difficulties with social and occupational function, the performance of mental tasks such as household financial management, and multidimensional tasks such as driving. Although data demonstrating an unequivocal link between cognitive decline and quality of life after critical illness are currently lacking, possibly due to Type II errors, there is a relationship emerging in other areas [31,32].

The aetiology of cognitive dysfunction is undoubtedly multifactorial. Possible contributing factors include hypoxaemia, the toxic cerebral effects of sepsis, systemic inflammation and drugs [33]. Many patients exhibit delirium whilst acutely unwell, although this has proved surprisingly hard to characterise [34]. The development of practical tools to identify and assess delirium will allow its relationship, if any, with post-discharge cognitive decline to be established [35].

The natural history of post–critical illness cognitive dysfunction is not understood. The limited data from studies that have examined patients at more than one time-point suggest that many, but certainly not all, patients exhibit some improvement [20,21]. Our preliminary data (unpublished) identify a significant improvement between 3 and 9 months, whereas depression and anxiety remained unchanged. Whether the improvement is genuine, rather than merely the effect of learning or improved vitality after convalescence improving test performance, is extremely difficult to know. Qualitatively, patients interviewed in clinic perceive that many aspects of their intellectual function have improved.

Practical aspects of cognitive function research after critical illness

Other than routine surgical cases, there is no possibility of obtaining baseline data. This presents an enormous challenge for interpretation. Test results must be compared with controls derived from population 'normals'. However, individuals volunteering to participate in studies to establish normal ranges for such tests may not represent the genuinely normal population. Investigators planning studies involving re-testing after an interval need to anticipate the effect of learning on test performance; this has been recognised for many tests in normal populations. However, learning is itself a cognitive function, further complicating interpretation. Additionally, the enthusiasm for intensive care survivors for voluntarily reattending hospitals is highly variable; the proportion of patients enrolled into studies also varies. This leads to the possibility of unpredictable enrollment bias; some patients may feel too ill or traumatised to attend the hospital, while others are back at work and simply do not wish to spend time attending. Estimates of the overall incidence of dysfunction derived from individual small studies must therefore be treated with caution. Finally, such studies are time-consuming, requiring substantial effort on behalf of both patient and investigator and have proved difficult to fund.

Why are the data from the surgical and anaesthetic literature important? Firstly, critical illness is frequently associated with surgery or post-surgical misadventure, and it is important to quantify the underlying effects of surgery and anaesthesia irrespective of the effects of added critical illness. Secondly, while this field has been extensively studied, there is considerable heterogeneity of experimental approach, making comparisons between studies extremely difficult. However, a consensus document has been published for cardiac surgery [36]. There is a danger of generating confusion in the critical care literature, and a strong argument exists for a similar consensus process. The various mainstream candidates for inclusion in a standardised test battery have been reviewed [37]. Although many of the tests that have been employed have not specifically been validated in the critically ill, such validation may prove an insuperable barrier.

The future research agenda

Given the small number and size of studies of cognitive dysfunction after critical illness, a substantial amount of simple descriptive work is still required. Thus it is imperative that the data generated from modest studies are comparable, so supporting the argument for a consensus strategy for test selection. The natural history in a variety of different clinical settings needs proper description. Such studies may eventually lead to insights into causation and thus interventions that may improve patient outcomes. However, this is a long way off. The relationship between cognitive dysfunction and quality of life has proved hard to demonstrate. This may suggest that there is no relationship, the studies were small exhibiting Type II errors, the tools are inadequate, or possibly a mixture of all three.

Clearly emerging is a picture of psychological difficulty and reduced quality of life for many patients during the recovery period after critical illness. Cognitive impairment is part of this. Our appreciation and our understanding of how to conduct research into it are only just beginning.

References

1. Pearsall J. *Oxford Concise English Dictionary*. Oxford: Oxford University Press, 1999.
2. Scragg P, Jones A, Fauvel N. Psychological problems following ICU treatment. *Anaesthesia* 2001;**56**:9–14.
3. Schelling G, Stoll C, Haller M, *et al*. Health-related quality of life and post-traumatic stress disorder in survivors of the acute respiratory distress syndrome. *Crit Care Med* 1998;**26**:651–9.
4. Pochard F, Lanore JJ, Bellivier F, *et al*. Subjective psychological status of severely ill patients discharged from mechanical ventilation. *Clin Intens Care* 1995;**6**:57–61.
5. Jones C, Griffiths RD, Macmillan RR, Palmer TEA. Psychological problems occurring after intensive care. *Br J Intens Care* 1994;**4**:46–53.
6. Tian ZM, Reis MD. Quality of life after intensive care with the sickness impact profile. *Intens Care Med* 1995;**21**:422–8.
7. Sukantarat KT, Brett SJ. Neuropsychological consequences of intensive care. In: Angus DC, Carlet J, eds. *Surviving Intensive Care (Update in Intensive Care and Emergency Medicine No. 39)*. Berlin: Springer-Verlag, 2003, pp. 51–61.
8. Dodds C, Allison J. Postoperative cognitive deficit in the elderly surgical patient. *Br J Anaesth* 1998;**81**:449–62.
9. Moller JT, Cluitmans P, Rasmussen LS, *et al*. Long-term postoperative cognitive dysfunction in the elderly: ISPOCD1 study. *Lancet* 1998;**351**:857–61.
10. Heyer EJ, Adams DC, Solomon RA, *et al*. Neuropsychometric changes in patients after carotid endarterectomy. *Stroke* 1998;**29**:1110–5.
11. Heyer EJ, Sharma R, Rampersad A, *et al*. A controlled prospective study of neuropsychological dysfunction following carotid endarterectomy. *Arch Neurol* 2002;**59**:217–22.

12. Roach GW, Kanchuger M, Mangano CM, *et al*. Adverse cerebral outcomes after coronary bypass surgery. *N Engl J Med* 1996;**335**:1857–63.

13. Kilminster S, Treasure T, McMillan T, Holt DW. Neuropsychological change and S-100 protein release in 130 unselected patients undergoing cardiac surgery. *Stroke* 1999;**30**:1869–74.

14. Newman MF, Kirchner JL, Philips-Bute B, *et al*. Longitudinal assessment of neurocognitive function after coronary artery bypass surgery. *N Engl J Med* 2001;**344**:395–402.

15. Van Dijk D, Keizer AM, Diephuis JC, Durand C, Vos LJ, Hijman R. Neuro-cognitive dysfunction after coronary artery bypass surgery: a systematic review. *J Thorac Cardiovasc Surg* 2000;**120**:632–9.

16. Zamvar V, Williams D, Hall J, *et al*. Assessment of neurocognitive impairment after off-pump and on-pump techniques for coronary artery bypass graft surgery: prospective randomised controlled trial. *Br Med J* 2002;**325**:1268–72.

17. Van Dijk D, Jansen EWL, Hijman R, *et al*. Cognitive outcome after off-pump and on-pump coronary artery bypass graft surgery. *JAMA* 2002;**287**:1405–12.

18. Diegeler A, Hirsch R, Schneider F, *et al*. Neuromonitoring and neurocognitive outcome in off-pump versus conventional coronary bypass operations. *Ann Thorac Surg* 2000;**69**:1162–6.

19. Stroobant N, Van Nooten G, Belleghem Y, Vingerhoets G. Short-term and long-term outcome in on-pump versus off-pump CABG. *Eur J Cardiothorac Surg* 2002;**22**:559–64.

20. Hopkins RO, Weaver LK, Pope D, Orme JF, Bigler ED, Larson-Lohr V. Neuropsychological sequelae and impaired health status in survivors of severe acute respiratory distress syndrome. *Am J Respir Crit Care Med* 1999;**160**:50–6.

21. Jackson JC, Hart RP, Gordon SM, *et al*. Six-month neurological outcome of medical intensive care unit patients. *Crit Care Med* 2003;**31**:1226–34.

22. Herridge MS, Cheung AM, Tansey CM, *et al*. One-year outcomes in survivors of the acute respiratory distress syndrome. *N Engl J Med* 2003;**348**:683–93.

23. Davidson TA, Caldwell ES, Curtis JR, Hudson LD, Steinberg KP. Reduced quality of life in survivors of acute respiratory distress syndrome compared with critically ill control patients. *JAMA* 1999;**281**:354–60.

24. Brooks R, Kerridge R, Hillman K, Bauman A, Daffurn K. Quality of life outcomes after intensive care: comparison with a community group. *Intens Care Med* 1997;**23**:581–6.

25. Kvale R, Flaatten H. Changes in health-related quality of life from 6 months to 2 years after discharge from intensive care. *Health Qual Life Outcomes* 2003;**1**:2–10.

26. Ridley SA, Chrispin PS, Scotton H, Rogers J, Lloyd D. Changes in quality of life after intensive care: comparison with normal data. *Anaesthesia* 1997;**52**:195–202.

27. Grant I, Heaton R, McSweeney A, Adams K, Timms R. Neuropsychological findings in patients with hypoxemic chronic obstructive pulmonary disease. *Arch Intern Med* 1982;**142**:1470–6.

28. Findley LJ, Barth JT, Powers C, Wilhoit SC, Boyd DG, Suratt PM. Cognitive impairment in patients with obstructive sleep apnoea and associated hypox-emia. *Chest* 1986;**90**:686–690.

29. Rothenhäusler H-B, Ehrentraut S, Stoll C, Schelling G, Kapfhammer H-P. The relationship between cognitive performance and employment and health status in long term-survivors of the acute respiratory distress syndrome: results of an exploratory study. *Gen Hosp Psychiatry* 2001;**23**:90–6.

30. Sukantarat KT, Williamson RCN, Burgess PJ, Brett SJ. Dysexecutive syn-drome after critical illness. *Am J Respir Crit Care Med* 2004;**169**:A628.

31. Newman MF, Grocott HP, Mathew JP, *et al.* Report of the sub-study assessing the impact of neurocognitive function on quality of life 5 years after cardiac surgery. *Stroke* 2001;**32**:2874–81.
32. Swearer JM. Cognitive function and quality of life. *Stroke* 2001;**32**:2880–1.
33. Papadopoulos MC, Davies DC, Moss RF, Tighe D, Bennett ED. Pathophysiology of septic encephalopathy: a review. *Crit Care Med* 2000;**28**:3019–24.
34. McNicoll L, Pisani MA, Zhang Y, Ely EW, Siegel MD, Inouye SK. Delirium in the intensive care unit: occurrence and clinical course in older patients. *J Am Geriatr Soc* 2003;**51**:591–8.
35. Ely EW, Inouye SK, Bernard GR, *et al.* Delirium in mechanically ventilated patients: validity and reliability of the confusion assessment method for the intensive care unit (CAM-ICU). *JAMA* 2001;**286**:2703–10.
36. Murkin JM, Newman SP, Stump DA, Blumenthal JA. Statement of consensus on assessment of neurobehavioural outcomes after cardiac surgery. *Ann Thorac Surg* 1995;**59**:1289–95.
37. Hopkins RO. How should we assess neuropsychological sequelae of critical illness. In: Angus DC, Carlet J, eds. *Surviving Intensive Care (Update in Intensive Care and Emergency Medicine No. 39)*. Berlin: Springer-Verlag, 2003, pp. 197–209.

8: The photo-diary and follow-up appointment on ICU: Giving back time to patients and relatives

CARL G BÄCKMAN, STEN M WALTHER

Introduction

Patients on the intensive care unit (ICU) often spend a great deal of their time either unconscious or heavily sedated. When they return from the zone between life and death, they are often confused when dreams and delusions are intertwined with reality and it is not always easy to distinguish between them.

The nurse said that those who were not tea-totallers would be thrown down a chute to a bath of hot water in the cellar. Next to the bath was a porter who fished out the dead bodies with a net. Since I've had a drink now and then, I was certain that I would end my days like this.

The distinction between dreams and reality may be even more difficult if well-meaning personnel say 'things are starting to look good now' when in fact the patient still has a tracheotomy, cannot breathe and can hardly turn in bed because of muscle weakness. This is especially so if the last memory is going to theatre for a cholecystectomy.

The only thing I could do was to blink and stare at the ceiling. I couldn't do anything. I couldn't fix my eyes on the wall. Yet I was clear in my head so time went so slowly. It was terrible not being able to move my arms and legs and it sounded strange when they said that I was getting better.

In our experience, very few patients dare to ask about their time on ICU. Questions are more often asked at the end of their hospital stay and frequently directed to the ward nurse who may have little knowledge about what happened on ICU. Similarly the ward medical staff who probably only saw the patient for a few minutes on the ICU round may be equally ignorant. The usual reply might be 'don't worry about what has been; you're on the way to recovery, so look to the future'.

Sometimes the patient is told that he or she was sedated and put on a ventilator (in Sweden we say 'in a ventilator'). This leads patients to believe that they were put into some sort of 'iron lung'. One patient told his relatives that he had been cared for in something that resembled a little submarine.

On several occasions, ward medical staff asked if a curious patient could possibly come to the ICU and see what it looked like. These patients asked strange questions and often found it hard to believe that they had ever been cared for on ICU since they had no recollection of their time there. Their idea of what the unit looked like often bore no resemblance to reality. Some patients were convinced that they had been cared for in another hospital in another town, or that they were journeying all the time they were unwell.

On asking patients about ICU just prior to discharge, the majority remembered little. Some patients could recall things but found it difficult or did not want to describe memories.

It was an upsetting time, all those unreal dreams, or was it death showing its face? It's not easy to understand all that is going on around you when you're drugged up to the eyeballs.

Initially we did not explore these memories further. One patient was later heard telling his friends that we had tried to kill him but that his relatives had forced us to give him medicine and as a result he had survived. This particular patient prompted us to help patients interpret and understand their experiences. It is not appropriate to return patients to physical health and then expect ward personnel to help them understand everything they went through during weeks of intensive care. Similarly this should not be left to the relatives who may have little chance of understanding all that is happening. In the early 1990s we received the following telephone call:

During the time my husband was on the ICU everything apart from getting him well again was of little interest. I went about daily chores as though in a trance, my thoughts were with him all the time even when I wasn't by his side and I could hardly sleep. The personnel were wonderful; they explained what they were doing and what was to be done and I thought I understood. Now, when I have him home and well again, he has asked me about what happened on the ICU and I have difficulty in explaining. He doesn't realise just how sick he was and when I tell him he was seriously ill with high fever, it's as though he cannot take it in. He just lies in bed and worries, sometimes he asks strange things and has even asked me if I came and visited him. I was there every day and we laughed and joked those last days on the ICU but he cannot remember anything about that. If we come up to ICU, can someone help me tell him about it? He cannot cope all that much but he's at his best around 10 o'clock, would that be OK?

Some patients are ashamed of their memories and feel guilty. By informing them that it is quite usual for patients to have delusions and nightmares after intensive care, it is possible for them to understand their experience.

Introduction of the photo-diary and follow-up appointment

Memory gaps from their time on ICU may contribute to patients' unreal delusions [1]. If there is no natural explanation, then people tend to search for answers and even invent them. Gaps in memory can be filled with semi-conscious recollection, which only partly represents the truth. Keeping a diary with photographs could fill these memory gaps with facts of what really happened on ICU. Together the staff and relatives can build up a record of important daily events and milestones during the patient's stay using coloured photographs and a written diary. The diary is written in a non-technical way for ease of understanding and can be read later at home in peace and quiet. Photographs are taken with the relatives' permission; they should be realistic but avoid nudity, which could embarrass the patient (Figure 8.1). We use a digital camera and print out the pictures on ICU.

Everyone involved with the patient, including relatives, can write in the diary but they are not obliged to; they do it because they realise how important it is for the patient and relatives to have a record of what happened. Each entry must be signed. It is important to give a genuine picture of how serious the situation is, otherwise it is difficult for the patient to see when improvement started. Contributors to the diary are instructed to avoid irrelevant information such as weather but to note daily routines

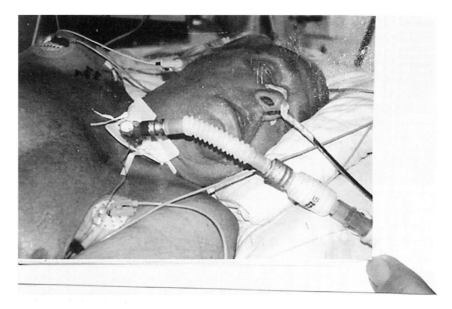

Figure 8.1 A sedated patient with a tracheotomy in the ICU.

and the patient's reactions. These are some typical examples picked from the same diary written by nurses and a physician:

You had difficulties in breathing so we had to help by putting a tube via the mouth into your windpipe and connect you to a ventilator. We put you to sleep first. Your circulation was very unstable and we had to give you a lot of blood and plasma. We also had to clean your blood with the help of a kidney machine (Friday 16th November).

You were more awake last night (this sounds stupid but we mean that you were more 'with it'). You make faces when we turn you on your side to nurse you so you are given extra pain relief. We can also see that you try to help a little, it isn't much but it makes us happy (night between Saturday and Sunday 26th November).

Hi Mary. It's I who received you when you came to the ICU and since then I've been involved in your treatment for a serious infection and its complications. You have been heavily sedated most of the time but today you're starting to wake up and certainly wondering what has happened since the 15th November when you came. Today I've told you about your first days here and the major operation on the 16th November where the right leg had to be amputated at the hip if you were to have any chance of surviving.

    Now things are starting to look better but it must be a great shock to wake up and find your right leg missing. I'll be coming back to talk to you about this in the days to come (27th November).

A relative wrote the following:

Good evening Nicke. Just now it's 10:30 in the evening and we've just said good-night to each other. It has been a quiet day. They've X-rayed your lungs and it seems that a part of the lung has collapsed. The nurse says that it's only a case of blowing more air into the lungs – a bagatelle. They're also going to X-ray your right arm to see how it looks under the plaster as well as your swollen left leg. You don't need so much morphine now. Madeleine misses you a lot and I know how she must feel being so far away while you're so poorly. Mum is sitting here and knitting you a red scarf, she says that it's difficult to express herself in words. One thing is for sure, we certainly couldn't hope for a finer mum. Even though you're covered in bruises you run the risk of getting even more if she carries on kissing your cheeks like she does. We miss you. Love Eva.

    The photo-diary is a tool that we create during the patient's time on ICU to use later in the rehabilitation process. Usually a few weeks after leaving the unit the patient and relatives are judged to be in a position to be able to absorb information, and so they are invited for a follow-up appointment. The photo-diary is then used as a guide to the events that took place. By giving the patient and relatives logical and chronological information based on fact as early as possible, they are better equipped to deal with their trauma. We believe that confrontation with reality is of benefit regardless of how negative the situation is as long as the individual is ready and not forced.

The object of the photographs, which are taken on all sorts of occasions (e.g. resting, being examined, having a visit, being nursed, mobilisation), is to give patients a more concrete understanding of how sick they have been. This prepares them for the long convalescence period to come so they understand that it will take many months and not just weeks before they are restored to normal life. Our aim is to give them realistic expectations and to encourage them to take responsibility for their rehabilitation at home. As soon as the patient leaves the ICU, the diary is handed over to the patient to continue so that the whole episode from ICU admission to hospital discharge is covered. The photographs are presented to the patient at the follow-up appointment since it is not suitable to see such pictures until they can properly be explained. Once explained, they are then inserted into designated spaces in the diary.

So far we have kept a diary for over 200 patients, and our experience is that a few minutes' writing in the diary each day, the photographs and the follow-up appointment all serve to fill any gaps that may have occurred in the patient's or relatives' memory of the time spent in hospital (Figure 8.2). It gives structure to the discussion at the follow-up appointment and often acts as a catalyst enabling the patient or relatives to ask questions that arise [2]. At first, the follow-up appointment was used only to complete the photo-diary. However, now it is an opportunity to make patients understand just how poorly they were and why it will take time before complete recovery is achieved. One goal is to enable the patient to understand and accept the limitations imposed by illness thereby providing encouragement to go on. The photo-diary also shows how much better patients have become since their ICU admission.

I thought that two pictures were horrible but I had to see them. Now I understand why doctors and nurses think that it's a wonder that I'm alive. I'll never complain about my scars again.

The follow-up appointment with patients and relatives is extremely valuable to ICU staff, allowing them to see the final results of their efforts and so increasing understanding and job satisfaction. Meeting former patients and their relatives has been rewarding and has allowed the opportunity to ask about their experiences.

Use of the photo-diary when a patient dies

Unfortunately about a quarter of the patients for whom we have kept a diary have died while still in hospital. These patients spent on average 3 weeks on ICU (Table 8.1). At the start we were hesitant in giving the relatives the diary, but as time passed we found that the diary helped mourning process. A questionnaire given to the relatives of 26 patients who died showed that in 6 cases the diary was regarded as invaluable,

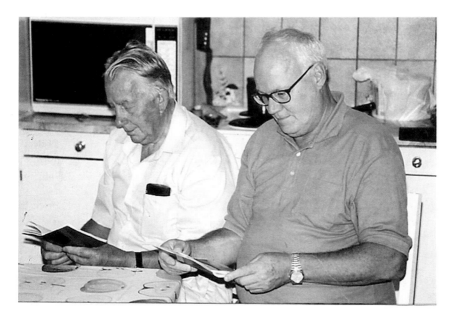

Figure 8.2 Two former patients reading each other's diary and sharing experiences of their time on ICU.

Table 8.1   Data of 26 patients with a diary who died

	Mean value (range) or number
Age (years)	65 (39–82)
Female patients	10
Time on ICU (days)	20.5 (2–56)
TISS[a] (points)	401 (74–928)
Time on ventilator (days)	16.5 (0.1–51)
APACHE II derived probability of death[b] (%)	46 (17–92)
Diagnosis	
Pneumonia	9
Abdominal surgery	6
Aortic aneurysm	3
Sepsis	3
Other	5

[a] Workload measured with the Therapeutic Intervention Scoring System (TISS).
[b] Illness severity assessed with the Acute Physiology and Chronic Health Evaluation II System (APACHE II).

very helpful in 11 and helpful in 5. Two relatives, who did not attend follow-up, said it was of no significance. The relatives of one patient refused to answer because of a family dispute after the patient died, and another relative simply did not want the diary. Even when it is a relative to the deceased involved, we still feel it best to hand over the diary at a follow-up appointment [3].

These are some extracts written by next of kin picked from three different diaries:

The diary has helped us in our mourning, we haven't had to explain to relatives and friends what Dad's last days on the ICU were like and they also found it helpful. It also feels good to be able to express one's sorrow in words, the thoughts we had and things we wanted to say to him. We felt it was important as relatives to be able to take part in Dad's 'everyday life' on the ICU and to be able to read what you nurses did with him when we weren't there. It warms our hearts to see how well you treat patients who lie heavily sedated; the respect you show is clearly seen in the diary. For us the diary has been nothing else but positive. (four daughters)

During the period following the loss of my friend I used to carry the diary with me wherever I went. If ever a question arose I always had something concrete to refer to. He was very proud of his diary and used to talk a lot about it during the time he lived after his time on the ICU. (a friend)

The diary has been a great comfort during my time of mourning. The diary, the occasional lit candle, a visit to the grave and the comfort of a good friend to talk to have helped me to go on. (husband)

Conclusion

The photo-diary and the follow-up appointment give back to the patient the time that was lost while on ICU. They also eases the pressure on relatives and friends who otherwise have to repeatedly explain events that they themselves only partly recall. There is an obligation to explain why and what has been done to patients who are not able to give consent. The photo-diary is a useful tool in this respect. The diary is inexpensive and together with a follow-up appointment provides an ideal means of looking back at what has happened. It also helps us detect any early signs of psychological distress, in which case it is easy to arrange a consultation with a psychiatrist. In this situation the diary can be an important factor in the treatment of both patient and relatives.

Acknowledgements

The Research Board of Vrinnevisjukhuset, Norrköping, supported this work. We are grateful to Peter Cox, MD for help with the linguistic revision.

References

1. Jones C, Griffiths RD, Humphris G. Disturbed memory and amnesia related to intensive care. *Memory* 2000;**8**:79–94.
2. Bäckman CG, Walther SM. Use of a personal diary written on the ICU during critical illness. *Intens Care Med* 2001;**27**:426–9.
3. Granger C, Shelly M. Bereavement care. In: Griffiths RD, Jones C, eds. *Intensive Care Aftercare*. Oxford: Butterworth-Heinemann. 2002, pp. 133–41.

9: Suffering and coping: the challenges for staff

CARL S WALDMANN

Introduction

Only recently have the psychological consequences of treatment on an intensive care unit (ICU) started to be investigated. Knowledge in this field is limited for patients but even less is known about the effects of stress on the staff.

When many of us started our intensive care medicine careers 18–20 years ago, we were appointed to jobs as ICU Directors; we took over from eminent people who often ran units single-handedly. Some made themselves always available and in spite of their commitment were often inadequately supported and eventually 'burnt out'. This term 'burn out' was the first many of us encountered in the psychological aspects of our stressful job. It has been widely publicised that burn out can also occur in the ICU nursing staff [1].

The medical profession has only recently taken the concept of work-related stress seriously and Hospital Trusts have now been advised to implement 'stress policies' based on a recent Health and Safety Executive publication [2].

What is work-related stress?

The Health and Safety Executive defines work-related stress as 'the adverse reaction people have to excessive pressures or other types of demand put on them' leading to the perception that the person cannot cope at a given time; this is also known as destructive stress. This is to be distinguished from the beneficial effects of reasonable pressure and challenge, which can give a 'buzz' and be stimulating enough to enhance performance (known as constructive stress). Even though not a disease itself, work-related stress can lead to ill health (Box 9.1).

Box 9.1 Ill health associated with work-related stress

- Heart disease
- Back pain
- Gastrointestinal disturbance
- Maladaptive behaviour in the form of addiction to caffeine, nicotine, alcohol and drugs
- Overt depression

Workplace stress is worse for the heart than gaining 40 lb weight or ageing 30 years because workers deal with such stress by smoking, drinking and 'slobbing out' (according to BBC News on 5 August 2003). Of course the concept of work-related stress is not new; concerns about the implications of work-related stress have been taken seriously in many other industries such as the aviation industry where methods to reduce work-related stress have been introduced in an attempt to reduce errors leading to accidents. It is interesting that the design of the cockpit for the Eurofighter has been influenced by a team from a department of psychology. The pilot's sweating, pulse rate and EEG are monitored and when there are signs of stress, the computer will take over the flying of the jet. It is accepted in this industry that 'information overload' whilst pulling several 'g' of centrifugal force can adversely affect the safety of the mission [3]. It seems that compared to industries such as aviation and sports (for top-level football referees [4]), the medical world is way behind in monitoring both physical and psychological stress. Error reduction in the healthcare industry is probably the major catalyst for trusts to implement a 'work-related stress policy'.

Implications of work-related stress

Ninety-four percent of doctors and nurses felt that stress was causing increased absenteeism and 30% felt stress had led to standards being lowered; 10% said it could have led to medical error (reported on the BBC News, 4 April 2001). Knowing that work-related stress can lead to ill health in staff and poorer outcome in patients, it is inconceivable that employers would not minimise this risk. According to the Health and Safety at Work Act 1974 [5] employers are legally required to take appropriate action to minimise the risk of their staff developing work-related stress, and furthermore they must take account of the risks of stress-related ill health as detailed in the *Management of Health and Safety at Work* regulations 1999 [6]. The main provisions of these regulations are summarised in Box 9.2.

Box 9.2 The main provisions of the Management of Health and Safety at Work regulations 1999 [6]

- Assess the risk
- Apply the principles of prevention
- Ensure employee's capability and provide training

There is also an economic argument for tackling work-related stress. Looking at absence due to illness, Health and Safety Executive estimates 6.5 million working days lost in the UK in 1995 due to work-related stress. This is an average of 16 days per person with work-related stress or £3.75 billion lost in productivity. Recent research has demonstrated the benefits of effective people management [7]. For instance job satisfaction and good human resource management structures underpin improved profitability and productivity. In particular, expenditure and emphasis on research and development have been shown to improve productivity by 6% and profitability by 8%. There is no doubt that adequate supervision of ICU nursing staff is essential for reduced turnover and absenteeism and improved patient outcomes [8].

Doctors

Doctors have long been considered at special risk [9,10] but relatively few studies have been undertaken [11,12]. These studies demonstrate psychiatric morbidity between 22% and 46%. A recent study performed on UK intensive care doctors [13] found that one out of three doctors appeared distressed and one in ten depressed. In comparison the average British worker has a lower chance (17.5%) of developing psychiatric problems according to a 1995 Household Panel Survey [14].

At an average age of 42 years, doctors have 20 years more to contribute to the NHS, so it would seem prudent for trusts to minimise the possibility of work-related stress by implementing advice from documents such as 'Improving Working Lives' [15] and complying with the European Working Time Directive. There is now an opportunity with the new consultant contract [16] to ensure the working week is properly controlled, monitored and appropriately rewarded. Doctors cost £232,000 to train and each lost working year of a consultant costs £30,000 in terms of training [17]. It is, therefore, vital that resources and treatments are available in the hospital's occupational health departments to detect and deal with maladaptive coping behaviour such as alcohol and drug abuse.

Individual doctors have access to the British Medical Association Stress Counselling Service [18] and the National Counselling Service for

---

Box 9.3 The recognised stressors for an ICU consultant

- Finding a bed when ICU is full
- Compromising standards when resources are short
- Treatment withdrawal
- Keeping up to date
- Fear of making the wrong decision or a mistake and being humiliated or taken to court
- Conflict with colleagues
- Worry about home life
- Long hours
- Car parking

Box 9.4 Consultant review processes

- Internal enquiry
- External Royal College review
- Coroner's inquest
- Court
- General Medical Council (sometimes 12 months or more later)

Sick Doctors [19]. For an ICU consultant the well-known stressors are listed in Box 9.3.

If a complaint is made against a consultant, the process that follows can cause havoc at work and at home. If suspended, the doctor may face financial hardship due to loss of private practice whilst waiting for the case to be considered. The consultant may have to go through and appear before a variety of processes and committees (Box 9.4).

Trainees

Trainees may have similar causes of stress as their consultant colleagues, but additional stressors may be important (Box 9.5).

Box 9.5 Stressors for trainees

- Dealing with sick children
- Ambulance/helicopter transfers
- Inability to find consultant
- Fear of disturbing consultant who may think it too trivial
- Asked to attend an 'inappropriate' resuscitation call
- Volume of work
- Appraisal
- Commuting because of training post rotations

Nursing staff

Reducing occupational stress in intensive care nursing staff has recently been the subject of a review [20], and interestingly has pointed to the issues of a noisy environment and bullying. Bullying and harassment at work have been reviewed recently [21]. Box 9.6 lists some common concerns.

Strategic decision-making

Stress and the need for adequate support also apply to those doctors and senior nurses entrusted with strategic decision-making. These individuals have to balance the needs of the patients and ICU staff against the available

Box 9.6 Common concerns of nursing staff

- Morale and organisational climate
- Insufficient staff
- Litigation and humiliation for mistakes
- Lack of recognition of workload
- Physical environment, noise pollution
- Security when going home after a late shift
- Unanticipated physician interference
- Death of a paediatric patient
- Dealing with relatives. Patients enter ICU in a biological crisis whereas the relatives are in a psychological crisis

resources. They must try and implement the recommendations of documents such as the Intensive Care Society's Standards Document, 'Critical to Success' (Audit Commission), Comprehensive Critical Care (Department of Health), National Institute for Clinical Excellence guidance on the use of ultrasound for CVP line placement [22,23,24,25]. For example, 30 doses of activated Protein C costs the same as seven extra nurses. If the seven extra ICU nurses are chosen, are they deployed to an outreach service or a follow-up clinic or an extra ICU bed?

Future directions

Helping staff cope with the challenges of running a critical care service and administering to the needs of critically ill patients can be dealt with by ensuring the service is adequately resourced, equipped and staffed for the expected workload. Adequate training and supervision of staff improves outcomes for patients and reduces work-related stress and absenteeism amongst the staff. As a recent Intensive Care Society publication demonstrates, there is a wide variation in the provision of critical care beds per 500 acute hospital beds throughout the UK [26]. Many ICUs are under-resourced and therefore it is highly likely that staff in these units will be at risk of developing work-related stress.

The Institute of Medicine (IOM) in the USA published a report in 2000: *To Err is Human: Building a Safer Health System*. This looked at issues around medical errors and how they could be prevented. The report estimates that up to 98,000 deaths are caused annually in the USA by medical error, making it the seventh leading cause of death [27].

Unsafe acts are like mosquitoes. You can try to swat them one at a time, but there will always be others to take their place. The only effective remedy is to drain the swamps in which they breed. In the case of errors and violations, the 'swamps' are equipment designs that promote operator error, bad communications, high workloads, budgetary and commercial pressures, procedures that necessitate their violation in order to get the job done, inadequate organisation, missing barriers and safeguards. [28]

Most errors are system-related rather than individual errors. In order to minimise errors and, in so doing, reduce one of the major causes of stress in medical staff working on ICU, the IOM report recommends the use of evidence-based medicine, electronic physician order entry systems and clinical decision support systems. In order to be effective, these recommendations need to be available at the point of care (i.e. at the bedside on a workstation). This means ICUs need to procure a clinical information system to implement these recommendations. Progress with this may soon be enforced in the USA following an initiative by a business

			PKK	CEC	CEC	CEC	ETM	ETM	CEC	CEC	MML	MML
HAEM	Hb	g/dL	10.10			9.40			9.20			9.00
	HCT	%			42.00		57.00	54.00		39.00	30.00	
	WBC	10^9/L	17.78			14.55			14.55			15.71
	RBC	10^12/L	3.2									
	MCV	fl										
	MCHC	g/dL										
	MCH	pg										
	RDW	%										
	Platelet Cnt	10^9/L				320			320			326
	NRBC	10^9/L										
COAG	APD	sec										
	APTR		1.30			1.30			1.40			1.03
	INR		0.98						1.04			1.40
		sec										
	TT	sec										
	Fibrinogen	mg/dL										
	FDP	ng/mL										
	Bleeding Time	min										
INFEC DX	Specimen Results											
Charted By			PKK	CEC	CEC	CEC	ETM	ETM	CEC	CEC	MML	MML

Figure 9.1 A transcription error caused by not linking the pathology service with the ICU clinical information system.

consortium known as the Leapfrog Group comprising major industrial firms such as General Electrics, General Motors, IBM and Boeing. The consortium will only recommend private medical care for their employees in an approved hospital if the hospital ICU has intensive-led ward rounds and where the initiatives of evidence-based medicine, electronic physician order entry systems and clinical decision support are practiced [29]. In the UK, progress at the moment is slow for ICUs without clinical information systems, as trusts will delay procurement of these systems whilst a national project for implementation of hospitalwide electronic patient record (EPR) takes shape. At present it is unclear what arrangements are being made with the EPR national project for data capture in the information-rich environment of the ICU [30].

Most trusts have 'island' solutions, that is, in the absence of a hospitalwide system they have isolated systems in the laboratory, maybe ICU and a Picture Archiving and Communication System (PACS) in radiology. With discrete systems that are not integrated with each other, mistakes are possible when data are transferred manually from the workstation receiving the laboratory results to the clinical information system (Figure 9.1)[31].

Conclusion

Work-related stress occurs commonly in ICU staff and can lead to physical illness due to maladaptive behaviour such as alcohol addiction. Trusts should ensure they implement Health and Safety Executive recommendations and have a stress policy. Adequate supervision of nursing staff may reduce the incidence of work-related stress and absenteeism and may improve staff retention. Provision of adequate resources as recommended in the *Intensive Care Society Standards Document*, the Audit Commission's report and *Comprehensive Critical Care* will help staff cope with the pressures of working on ICU. Reducing the possibility of medical errors by the use of health informatics is a key development for the future.

References

1. Appleyard N, Langan S. Human resources and education. In: Goldhill D, Withington S, eds. *Textbook of Intensive Care*. London: Chapman & Hall, 1997, p. 766.
2. Health and Safety Executive. *Tackling Work-related Stress*. London: Health and Safety Executive (HSE), 2001.
3. Taylor RM, Finnie SE. The cognitive cockpit: operational requirement and technical challenge. In: McCabe P, Hanson M A, Robertson S, eds. *Contemporary Ergonomics* London: Taylor and Francis, 2000, pp. 55–9.
4. D'Ottavio S, Catagna C. Physiological load imposed on elite soccer referees during actual match play. *J Sports Med and Phys Fitness* 2001;**41**:27–32.
5. Her Majesty's Stationery Office. Health and Safety at Work Act 1974. London: Her Majesty's Stationery Office (HMSO), 1974.

6. Management of Health and Safety at Work Regulations 1999. Approved code of practice and guidance. Sudbury: Health and Safety Executive, 2000.

7. Patterson MG, West MA, Lawthom R, Nickell S. Impact of people management practices on business performance. London: Institute of Personnel and Development (ISBN 0852927258), 1997;**22**:ix–xi.

8. Temple C, Shelly M. Clinical supervision: supporting staff and raising standards. In: Griffith RG, Jones C, eds. *Intensive Care Aftercare*. Oxford: Butterworth-Heinemann, 2002, pp. 156–64.

9. Smith R. All doctors are problem doctors. *Br Med J* 1997;**314**:841–2.

10. Firth-Cozens J. Hours, sleep, teamwork and success. *Br Med J* 1998;**317**:1335–6.

11. Caplan RP. Stress, anxiety and depression in hospital consultants, general practitioners and senior health service managers. *Br Med J* 1994;**309**:1261–3.

12. Blenkin H, Deary IJ, Wood RA, Zeally HE, Agius RM. Stress in NHS consultants. *Br Med J* 1995;**310**:534.

13. Coomber S, Todd C, Park G, Baxter P, Firth-Cozens J, Shore S. Stress in UK intensive care doctors. *Br J Anaesth* 2002;**89**:873–81.

14. British Household Panel Survey 1993–4. UK Data Archive for the 1995 Household Panel Survey. Colchester Institute for Social and Economic Research, 2001. www.irc.essex.ac.uk/bhps

15. Department of Health. *Improving Working Lives*. London: Department of Health, 2002.

16. Ridley S. The new contract. *J Intens Care Soc* 2004;**5**:36.

17. Netten A, Knight J, Dennet J, Coolley R, Slight A. A 'Ready Reckoner' for staff costs in the NHS. Canterbury: Personal Social Services Research Unit, 2000;**1**:79.

18. BMA Stress Counselling Service. *BMJ News* 1996;**6 July**:313.

19. Davies RH. Junior doctors and stress. *Lancet* 1998;**352**:1780.

20. Corr M. Reducing occupational stress in intensive care. *Nurs Crit Care* 2000;**5**:76–80.

21. Barrett G. Bullying and harassment at work: time to take action. *J Neonat Nurs* 2004;**10**:59–61.

22. Intensive Care Society. *Standards for Intensive Care Units*. London: Intensive Care Society, 1997.

23. Audit Commission. *Critical to Success*. The place of efficient and effective critical care services within the acute hospital. London: Audit Commission Publications, 1999.

24. Department of Health. *Comprehensive Critical Care*: a review of adult critical care services. London: Department of Health, 2000.

25. National Institute of Clinical Excellence. Guidance on the use of ultrasound locating devices for placing central venous catheters. *Technology Appraisal Guidance* No. 49. London: National Institute of Clinical Excellence, 2002.

26. Intensive Care Society. *Critical Insight*. An Intensive Care Society (ICS) introduction to UK adult critical care services 2003. London: Intensive Care Society, 2003.

27. Kohn LT, Corrigan JM, Donaldson M. *To Err Is Human: Building a Safer Health System*. Committee on Quality of Healthcare in America, Institute of Medicine. Washington, DC: National Academy Press, 2000.

28. Reason JT. Though ecologically unsound, the analogy is apt. In: Bogner MS. Hillsdale, eds. *Foreword to Human Error in Medicine*. Hillsdale NJ: Lawrence Erlbaum Association, 1994.

29. Martinez B. Business consortium to launch effort seeking higher standards at hospitals. *Wall St J* 2000;**15 Nov**:A3.

30. Kapila A. Letter to the Editor. *J Intens Care Soc* 2004;**5**:39.

31. Imhoff M, Waldmann C. *Health Informatics*. Brussels: European Society of Intensive Care Medicine, 2003.

Index

INDEX